What I Wish I Knew...

Success for your Bariatric Life

Dr. Jeanie Woolledge, PhD, LPC

Copyright 2024 by Dr. Jeanie Woolledge, PhD, LPC

All rights reserved. No part of this book may be reproduced or transmitted in any form or by any means, electronic or mechanical, including photocopying, recording or by any information storage and retrieval system, without the written permission of the Publisher, where permitted by law.

ISBN: 9-781304-981394

Printed in the United States of America

Books by Dr. Jeanie Woolledge, PhD, LPC
　　　Aka J Marie:
LIVES OF DECEPTION
LIVES OF TRAGEDY AND HOPE
SOPHIE, NO!
SOPHIE, NO! ACTIVITY BOOK
SOPHIE GETS A BABY SISTER
SOUTHERN FAMILY COOKBOOK
YOU ARE AMAZING!

To my family, for their unwavering love and support. To the bariatric community…may we all go through the journey together. To all those who suffer and those who still suffer in silence.

To God, the true one that has all the answers, thank you for using me as I am just the vessel.

Table of Contents

Foreword 6

Introduction 8

Acronyms 14

Part I - Mental Wellness 20

    Chapter 1 - Why Do You Eat? 22

        Mental Part 25

        Emotional Eating 28

        Emotional Eating Tips 41

        Relationship with Food 44

        Stress Eating 54

    Chapter 2 - Healing Your Mind 58

        Self-Esteem 65

        Shame 72

        Body Image 75

        Coping Skills 82

        Letting Go 93

        Love Thyself 98

        Positive Affirmations 101

        Mindfulness 109

    Chapter 3 - Social Changes 117

- Relationships 119
- Boundaries 123
- Support 128
- Chapter 4 - Mental Health Issues 132
  - Anxiety 135
  - Depression 138
  - Eating Disorders 142
  - Body Dysmorphia 147
  - Transfer Addictions 150
  - Trauma 150
  - PTSD 158
  - Triggers 161
- Part II - Living the Bariatric Life 170
  - Chapter 5 - Pre-Surgery 172
    - Pre-op Challenges 181
    - Advice 183
    - Things to Do 187
    - Bring to the Hospital 189
    - Goals 192
    - Complications 195
  - Chapter 6 - Post-Surgery 199
    - Post-op Diet 206

- Rules 209
- Vitamins 214
- Water 217
- Food and Drinks 219

Chapter 7 - Living in Wellness 221
- The Process 224
- Life after Bariatric Surgery 226
- Exercise 230
- Maintenance 241

Chapter 8 - Lifestyle Benefits 243
- NSV's 248
- Rewards 253
- Positives 257
- Gratitude 259
- Realizations 263

Chapter 9 - Physical Benefits 265
- Weight Loss 268
- Looks Change 271
- Health 274

Chapter 10 - Struggles 277
- Struggles 283
- Body Side Effects 285

Pain 287

Bowels 289

Bones...291

Regrets...293

Burnout..296

Skin 300

Losing too much Weight 303

Grazing..306

Dumping 308

Regain..310

Back to Basics 315

Part III - BONUS: What I am looking forward to after weight loss..320

References..328

Foreword

All bariatric surgeons *should* make education a high priority for patients who are considering weight loss surgery. We try to make sure that every patient is aware not only of the risks and benefits of this surgery, but also of the lifestyle changes and mental adjustments that would insure a *high* degree of success as a primary outcome. And as the instructors, we can only parrot back to our patients what we have learned from those who have actually undergone these procedures.

Adequate preoperative education is a lot to absorb. And patients come away with different levels of completeness of understanding and preparation. And that is where *this* book can have its most significant impact.

The decision to undergo weight loss surgery is one of the biggest choices a person can make. This choice will have tremendous impact on the rest of their life. It is on the scale of "who should I marry?" or "what career path do I choose?" or "am I ready to start a family?" It is NOT similar to "should I get a new haircut?" or "where should I go on vacation?"

Yet, as a bariatric surgeon, I see people making this decision with the same lack of forethought and preparation every day. They come to my office and say, "I just want that 'make me skinny' surgery" or "my girlfriend had the surgery, and she looks great, so sign me up." These individuals are in for a *rude* awakening, and not very likely to succeed on this complex journey of the "bariatric life." It is NOT the "easy way out!"

Having weight loss surgery is *not* like having a hernia repair, or your gallbladder removed. In these cases, it is more of a necessity for your physical body and its continued function. Weight loss surgery is a highly complex and drastic metabolic alteration, which involves not only your physical body, *but* also your emotional sensibilities and your deepest personal relationships. Gaining insight into this process from the beginning is *essential and critical* to successful outcomes.

Dr. Jeanie Woolledge has provided a comprehensive and detailed resource for prospective weight loss patients, giving them an in-depth examination of what they need to know at the beginning (pre-surgery), and what they can expect throughout this journey (post-surgery). As one of my most successful bariatric surgery patients, she has a PhD in counseling studies, and is a Licensed Professional Counselor. She also executes bariatric psychological evaluations. Dr. Woolledge has authored a *highly* valuable tool based not only on her personal experience with surgical weight loss but has incorporated her expertise and testimony from many others who have confirmed and complemented her understanding of this complex transformation through the bariatric life.

Her approach appeals to patients as well as surgical teams who are looking for a more robust manual to equip patients with the information they need in a narrative as well as a bullet point format. Questions posed allow patients to self-reflect and become more aware.

This book *should* be required reading for anyone who is entering this path, and a ready resource throughout their journey. It *should* be included in the pre-surgery information at all bariatric surgeon's offices.

David C. Treen, Jr, MD, FACS, FASMBS
Founder and CEO, Surgical Clinic of Louisiana
MBSAQIP Certified Bariatric Surgery Center of Excellence

Introduction

You're thinking about getting bariatric surgery or have already had the surgery. *Good news!* This book will address pre-op, post-op and more!! Here you will find the keys to a *successful* bariatric life. In addition, you will also find responses from other bariatric patients during all phases of their journey. Learning from them will assist you to better prepare yourself and teach you how to live a successful bariatric life.

Bariatric surgery is one of the most *life-changing* decisions of your life. Having bariatric surgery is both drastic and life-altering. No matter where you are in the journey, you will face challenges. Use this book for reference, support, and self-reflection during your bariatric lifetime. The tools and discoveries you will find will aid you to be successful in the ups and downs of bariatric life.

Experiencing many emotions such as fear, excitement, hope, or relief is common. But one thing is for sure. You want to embark upon your bariatric surgery journey loaded with tools and knowledge to *ensure* complete success.

Your surgical team will guide you and give you all you need to succeed physically. Your surgeon, who's done hundreds, or thousands of bariatric surgeries will be the expert you need to rely on during the pre-surgery, surgery, and post-surgery process. A bariatric dietician will give you all the tools you need to educate you on what you can eat, as well as the new rules to live by after bariatric surgery. This book, *"What I wish I Knew"* will fill in the *missing pieces* that addresses the mental and emotional part. This very important part has been the *missing link* to bariatric surgery success.

Why is it we hear about bariatric surgery failures? People preparing for bariatric surgery are asking questions like, "When can I drink alcohol again; have Diet Coke again, bread, rice, etc." This is *not* a good way to go into surgery or live post-op. Change your mindset to accept that you will *not* be able to eat or drink some of the very things that were unhealthy for you and caused you to be right where you are now. Fill your mindset with positive thoughts, good coping skills, and a dedication to whatever you have to do to guarantee a *lifetime of success!*

GOOD LUCK!!

DISCLAIMER: Not *all* bariatric patients will experience *everything* that is expressed in this book, *What I Wish I Knew*. Your regimen may or may not be different based on your bariatric surgical team. Please follow <u>YOUR</u> doctor's advice and follow <u>YOUR</u> plan.

Any questions or concerns should be asked of your bariatric team. Do *not* rely on this book as your only source of information.

Opinions expressed in this book may be from the bariatric community but does *not* represent the bariatric community as a whole.

Acronyms

AL – Arm Lift (Brachioplasty)

Aunt Flo – Menstruation Cycle/Period

BA – Breast Augmentation

BBL – Brazilian Butt Lift

BCP – Birth Control Pills

BL – Breast Lift

BM – Bowel Movement

BMI – Body Mass Index

BP – Blood Pressure

BPD – Biliopancreatic Diversion

BR – Breast Reconstruction

BTW – By the Way

CPAP – Continuous Positive Airway Pressure

CRAP – Carbonated drinks, Refined Sugar, Artificial & Processed foods

CW – Current Weight

DS – Duodenal Switch

EGD - Endoscopy

EKG - Electrocardiogram

ESG – Endoscopic Sleeve Gastroplasty

EWL – Excess Weight Loss or Expected Weight Loss

FBL – Full Body Lift

FDL – Fleur de lis (Ext. Tummy Tuck)

FF – Fat Free

FL – Facelift (Rhytidectomy)

F2FF/FTF – Face-to-Face Friday or Face-to-Face

FTW – For the Win or Faith that Works

FUPA – Fatty Upper Pubic Area

FYI – For Your Information

GERD – Gastroesophageal Reflux Disease

GF – Gluten Free

GI - Gastrointestinal

GP – General Practitioner

GPS – God Provides Strength

GW – Goal Weight

HC – Horrible Constipation

HW – Highest Weight

IDK – I don't know

IGB – Intragastric Balloon

IMHO – In my honest (or humble) Opinion

IMO – In My Opinion

LAP BAND - Laparoscopic Adjustable Gastric Band

LIPO – Liposuction

LSG – Laparoscopic Sleeve Gastrectomy

LW – Lowest Weight

LMK – Let me know

MGB – Mini Gastric Bypass

MM – Motivation Monday

MOM – Milk of Magnesia

MR – Muscle Repair

NL – Neck Lift (Lower Rhytidectomy)

NP – No Problem

NSAIDS – Non-Steroidal Anti-Inflammatory Drug

NSV – Non-scale Victory

NUT – Nutritionist/Dietician

OSA – Obstructive Sleep Apnea

Onederland – Weight in the 100's

PANNI – Panniculectomy

PCOS – Poly-Cystic Ovarian Syndrome

PCP – Primary Care Physician

PITA – Pain in the A$$

PO – Pre-Operative or Post-Operative

PPI – Proton Pump Inhibitors

PS – Plastic Surgeon

RD – Reset Diet

RNY – Roux-en-Y (Roux-en-Y Gastric Bypass

RW – Regained Weight

SF – Sugar Free

Stalls – This refers to an extended period when you are not making any progress on your weight loss efforts. It is a weight loss plateau where you are unable to lose any more weight.

Surgiversary – Surgical Anniversary

SW – Surgery Weight or Starting Weight

TBT – Throwback Tuesday or Thursday

TBWL – Total Body Weight Loss

TIA – Thanks in Advance

TICU – This is Completely Unacceptable (As spoken in Dr. Nowzaradan's voice)

TL – Thigh Lift

TLDR – Too Long Didn't Read

TMI – Too Much Information

TT – Tummy Tuck (Abdominoplasty)

Twoderville – Weight in the 200's

TY – Thank you

VBG – Vertical Banded Gastroplasty

VIT – Vitamins

VSG – Vertical Sleeve Gastrectomy (Gastric Sleeve Surgery)

WLS -Weight Loss Surgery

WTG – Way to Go!

YW – You're Welcome

Part I - Mental Wellness

Chapter 1

Why Do You Eat?

"Your words have so much power. Every day, if you tell yourself 'I love you,' if you give yourself one word of validation, it will change your mind."
— Ashley Graham

What some of the bariatric community has said:

1. Stalls are so frustrating.
2. How hard breaking up with food would be.
3. No longer enjoy eating like you used to.
4. Know your strengths and weaknesses.
5. I miss the fat girl.
6. The eyes are bigger than the stomach.
7. Bariatric surgery did nothing to help my thinking.
8. More mental and emotional strength was needed.
9. Mental acceptance is hard.

10. Mental health needs to be a priority.
11. You will mourn food and the old you.
12. Moods can swing from anger to depression.
13. Head hunger = madness.
14. Figure out what I'm eating over first.
15. I should have dealt with emotional eating.
16. Will change your relationship with food.
17. My mental struggle is hard as I struggle every day.
18. We can't forget about the mental part that got us here in the first place.
19. I went back to my old habits of emotional eating.
20. I feel so overwhelmed with my thoughts right now.
21. Feeling a little depressed before I start my pre-op diet.
22. When I reached onederland and reached my goal I felt so emotional.
23. Having a therapist both pre- and post-op was crucial.

24. I was pretty stable before surgery and now I find it difficult emotionally to process my emotions.
25. We don't have to "diet" to change our relationship with food.
26. Food used to be my best friend. Now it terrifies me.
27. I still love food, just get full very fast.
28. This foodie realized that after surgery I wasn't not going to love food again.
29. Food was something my family bonded over every night since my dad was a chef.
30. I turn to food when I'm stressed.
31. If only I could eliminate stress in my life.
32. I have found other options to eating when I'm stressed.

Mental Part

"The hardest work was changing the insides, getting to the mental place where I know I'm gonna be okay and then the weight was just, kinda, a lot easier. At a certain point, it just started coming off."

— Shannon Beador,
The Real Housewives of Orange County

Take control of your mental state and you *will* succeed! Get into therapy to address the underlying issues *before* surgery! Bariatric surgery is physically and mentally hard, so to assure your success, be more prepared. Weight loss is 90% diet, but your brain can interfere with you equally as much. If you have the surgery and *still* have issues with eating and emotions and you are *still* making poor food choices, a mindset change needs to happen.

Realistically, people should not depend on *just* using the tool given during bariatric surgery. It's only a tool, *not* a magic wand! Your mental thoughts and feelings play a *huge* part in your successful journey.

Deep down you know *exactly* what you're capable of. You *must* be willing to let go of the bad habits, old mindset, things, and situations that are standing in the way of your success.

Eating over your emotions is *no* longer an option after bariatric surgery. You won't be able to turn to food for comfort and have long-term success. The mental struggle is *real*. It was real *before* surgery and it's even *more* real after surgery. Know this going in and be prepared. Learn healthy coping skills to turn to instead of food.

7 Bariatric Truths that will Change your Mindset
1. Not everyone will support you.
2. Comparison will rob you of joy.
3. Losing weight slower doesn't = Failure.
4. Taking your vitamins is for life.
5. You don't have to lose weight every week to be successful.
6. There are no "good" or "bad" foods.

7. Healing your relationship with food takes effort, time, and self-compassion.

What mental struggles do you have?

_____

_____

_____

What are some of the things you can do without turning to food for comfort?

_____

_____

_____

Emotional Eating

Stop trying to fill the emptiness inside you with food.

When you eat in *response* to an emotion or feeling, emotional eating occurs. You aim to make yourself feel better by *trying* to fill emotional needs, rather than your stomach. Emotional eating can be over good or bad feelings. Think about the memories you had growing up surrounding food. Now think about times you are triggered, and you want to turn to food.

Unfortunately, emotional eating doesn't *fix* emotional problems. In fact, it usually makes you feel *worse*. Afterwards, the original emotional problem still remains.

Thoughts that go along with emotional eating is that eating this food will make you feel better and give you comfort. But it is *only* temporary. Soon will begin the cycle of guilt, then eating more food and then remorse. This vicious cycle can lead to thoughts of being a failure or even depression.

Emotions play a *huge* part in your eating habits. Some people binge when they're emotional, and they never realize it because they have trouble identifying what they are feeling at the moment.

It's not uncommon to see overweight people have severe emotional issues, and their efforts to cope include turning to food. Often those with high anxiety may turn to pizza, chips, and other carbohydrate-laden foods. The same principle causes someone to drink alcohol, use substances, or turn to any addiction.

Emotional eating drives people to use food to *numb* the pain. Unfortunately, it only works for a short time and is not a permanent solution. Additionally, counseling can help you see the need to control your eating habits and get to the core of your need to overeat. *Before* bariatric surgery is the time to address these important issues.

Emotional hunger is often used a way for connection, empathy, and compassion. The physical means of food will never fill these emotional needs. When you have unhealthy thoughts, it can be referred as "Stinkin' Thinkin'." These thoughts can cause you to make bad decisions that you may regret. Always *think* before you act. Going into autopilot mode can be the culprit towards unhealthy eating habits and actions.

But how do you tell the difference between emotional hunger and physical hunger? Do you turn to food when stressed? Are you hungry enough to eat an apple? If not, then you're probably not *truly* hungry. Rather, you are bored or seeking emotional support of some kind. You usually turn to food for comfort, stress relief, or to reward yourself by choosing unhealthy foods.

Emotional Eating Cycle

The emotional eating cycle begins with some emotion or something that happens to upset or trigger you. Suddenly you feel an overwhelming urge to eat.

You eat *more* than you know you should and feel guilty and powerless over food.

Occasionally, using food as a pick-me-up, a reward, or to celebrate isn't necessarily a bad thing. But when eating is your *primary* emotional coping mechanism—when your first impulse is to open the refrigerator whenever you're stressed, upset, angry, lonely, exhausted, or bored—you get stuck in an unhealthy cycle where the real feelings or problems are never addressed.

Emotional hunger *cannot* be filled with food. Eating may feel good in the moment, but the feelings that triggered the eating are still there, just buried temporarily. And then you often feel worse than you did before because of the unnecessary calories you've just consumed. Regrets begin and you beat yourself up for messing up and not having more willpower.

Intensifying the problem, you stop learning healthier ways to deal with your emotions, you have a harder and harder time controlling your weight, and you feel increasingly powerless over food and your feelings. But no matter how powerless you feel over food and your feelings, it is *possible* to make a positive change. You can learn healthier ways to deal with your emotions, avoid triggers, conquer cravings, and finally put a stop to emotional eating by learning new healthy coping skills.

Most emotional eaters feel powerless over their food cravings. When the urge to eat hits, it's all you can think about. There is an almost unbearable tension that demands to be fed, right now! Because you've tried to resist in the past and failed, you believe that your willpower just isn't up to par. But the *truth* is that you have more power over your cravings than you think.

Emotional Hunger vs. Physical Hunger

Learning how to distinguish between emotional and physical hunger will allow you to become free from the cycle of emotional eating. This might be difficult especially if you regularly use food to deal with your feelings. Look for clues to distinguish emotional hunger from physical hunger.

Emotional Hunger	Physical Hunger
Not satisfied with a full stomach	Satisfied when full
Comes on quickly	Comes on gradually
Craves certain comfort foods	Many foods sound good
Want to be satisfied instantly	Can wait
Triggers feelings of shame, powerlessness, and guilt	Don't feel bad about yourself

Common Causes of Emotional Eating

Stress. Do you ever notice how stress makes you hungry? It's not just in your mind. When stress is chronic, as it so often is in your chaotic, fast-paced world, your body produces high levels of the stress hormone, *cortisol*. Cortisol triggers cravings for salty, sweet, and fried foods—foods that give you a burst of energy and pleasure. The more uncontrolled stress in your life, the more likely you are to turn to unhealthy food for emotional relief.

Numbing Emotions. Eating can be a way to temporarily silence or *stuff down* uncomfortable emotions, including anger, fear, sadness, anxiety, loneliness, resentment, and shame. While you're numbing yourself with food, you can avoid the difficult emotions you'd rather not feel. The thought of not wanting to feel the pain of the emotions can lead to numbing.

Boredom or Feelings of Emptiness. Do you ever eat simply to give yourself something to do, to relieve boredom, or as a way to fill a void in your life? You feel unfulfilled and empty, and food is a way to occupy your mouth and your time. In the moment, it fills you up and distracts you from underlying feelings of purposelessness, loneliness, and dissatisfaction with your life.

Childhood Habits. Think back to your childhood memories of food. Did your parents reward good behavior with ice cream, take you out for pizza when you got a good report card, or serve you sweets when you were feeling sad? These habits can often carry over into adulthood. Or your eating may be driven by nostalgia—for cherished memories of grilling burgers in the backyard with your dad or baking and eating cookies with your mom.

Social Influences. Getting together with other people for a meal is a great way to relieve stress, but it can also lead to overeating. It's *easy* to overindulge simply because the food is there or because everyone else is eating. You may also overeat in social situations out of nervousness or social anxiety. Or perhaps your family or circle of friends encourage you to overeat or just take a taste, and it's easier to go along with the group.

Are you an Emotional Eater?

EMOTIONAL EATER QUESTIONNAIRE (EEQ)

Put the score next to the question: Never – 0 Sometimes – 1 Generally – 2 Always – 3

1. ___ Does the weight scales have a great power over you? Can they change your mood?

2. ___ Do you crave specific foods?

3. ___ Is it difficult for you to stop eating sweets, especially chocolate?

4. ___ Do you have problems controlling the amount of certain types of foods you eat?

5. ___ Do you eat when you're stressed, angry, or bored?

6. ___ Do you eat more of your favorite food and with less control when you are alone?

7. ___ Do you feel guilty when eating "forbidden foods," like sweets or snacks?

8. ___ Do you feel less control over your diet when you are tired after work at night?

9. ___ When you overeat while on a diet, do you give up and start eating without control, particularly food that you think is fattening?

10. ___ How often do you feel food controls you, rather than you controlling food?

Total Score: ____

0-5 – You are a *non-emotional eater*. Your emotions have little or nothing to do in your eating behavior. You are a person with great stability with respect to your eating behavior. You eat when you feel hungry, regardless of external factors or emotions.

6-10 – You are a *low emotional eater*. It is rare you solve your problems with food. However, you feel that certain foods affect your will.

11-20 – You are an *emotional eater*. Your responses indicate that to some extent your emotions influence your diet. Feelings and mood in some moments of your life determine how much and how you eat.

21-30 – You are a *very emotional eater*. If you're not careful, food will control your life. Your feelings and emotions constantly rotate around your food.

Check all that apply:

- ☐ Do you eat when you're not hungry? Or when you are sad, angry, lonely, or bored?
- ☐ Have you ever eaten past the point of being full?
- ☐ Do you open your pantry or refrigerator and just stare inside?
- ☐ Do you recognize when you are emotional or mindlessly eat while watching TV?
- ☐ Can you stop once you eat a few chips?
- ☐ Or can you leave a half of a candy bar for later?
- ☐ Do you turn to food for comfort, companionship, or just to feel better?
- ☐ Do you have your "special" love foods? The kind that brings you right back to your childhood.

- ☐ Do you have remorse after a binge and swear never to do that again?
- ☐ Do you eat in secret?
- ☐ Do you eat more when you're feeling stressed?
- ☐ Do you eat to feel better?
- ☐ Do you reward yourself with food?
- ☐ Do you eat when you're not hungry or when you're full?
- ☐ Do you eat to calm and soothe yourself when you're sad, mad, bored, or anxious?
- ☐ Do you regularly eat until you've stuffed yourself?
- ☐ Do you feel powerless or out of control around food?
- ☐ Does food make you feel safe?
- ☐ Do you feel like food is a friend?
- ☐ When you are having a bad day, do you stop for your favorite foods?
- ☐ Or do you stop at many fast-food places to get your favorites at each?

- [ ] Do you hide the wrappers? Or throw them away before you get home?
- [ ] Have you ever thrown foods away only to get them out again and eat them?
- [ ] Do you belong to the "clean your plate" club?
- [ ] Were you told there were starving children in Africa with no food?
- [ ] Were you given the option to eat or starve?

YOU ARE NOT ALONE!! YOU'RE PROBABLY AN EMOTIONAL EATER!!

Emotional Eating Tips

"Those who dare to fail miserably can achieve greatly."
— John F. Kennedy

Instead of turning to food to feel better, relieve stress, or feed your feelings, use these emotional eating tips:

- **Log your Food Daily.** In addition to putting down what you're eating, identify what is going on and how are you feeling.
- **Find Other Ways to Satisfy your Emotions.** Instead of eating over your emotions, develop a list of other things you can do. Do you have hobbies, activities, or friends that can help out?
- **Evaluate your Current Situation.**
    1. Are you hungry or just want to eat?
    2. Are you eating slower so you can identify if you are really full?
    3. Are you craving comfort food?

4. Can you do your hobbies or interests instead of eating?
5. Are you triggered?
6. Can you stop and think before you eat?
7. Do you remember that emotional eating doesn't fix emotional problems.
8. Can you turn to your support system for help?

Overcoming Emotional Eating

1. **What is your mood?**

   Learn to identify how you are feeling that makes you want to turn to food. Keep a journal and when tempted write about it so you can see if you are triggered.

2. **Wait it out.**

   Sometimes if you just sit with the feelings it will subside. Don't turn to food out of impulse. Wait it out or turn to healthy coping skills instead of eating.

3. **Turn to healthy coping skills.**

   Have a list available of activities or things you can do instead of eat. Remove yourself from your current situation. Try drinking some water. Sometimes hunger masks as thirst.

Relationship with Food

"There is no elevator to success. You have to take the stairs."
— Zig Ziglar

By exploring your history and relationship with food, you will see how that plays an important part of your journey so far. It's not just because you *love* to eat that brings you here. How food was handled growing up plays a *very* important foundational role. If your family emotionally used food, it would condition you to do the same. After all, you learn what you live. It is *critical* to replace unhealthy coping skills to truly be successful with your bariatric surgery life.

Food is neither "good" or "bad," "clean" or "not clean." This type of thinking sets you up for feeling *guilt* when you overeat certain food and develops an unhealthy relationship with food. Change your mindset to look at food as "healthy" or "unhealthy." What is unhealthy for you may be *different* than what is unhealthy for others. It's about *choice*. Every time you eat, you make a choice of what type of food you eat.

Learn ways to reward yourself with non-food options. Rewards are *good* and should be incorporated into your bariatric life. Choose healthy ways to celebrate.

Don't get overly hungry. Slow down when you eat. Plan and prepare what you are going to eat for the meal or day. *Planning* is key to be successful. Never open the refrigerator and say, "Now what?"

When you have a slip or eat something unhealthy, *don't* beat yourself up. Dust your knees off and start again. If you stay stuck in regret or remorse, the cycle of overeating can start. No one is perfect. It's not about how many times you fall. It's about how many times you pick yourself *up*.

Let's look at some of the ways that brought you to this important decision to have bariatric surgery, by examining your history and relationship with food.

Growing up, what role did food/overeating play in your family?

_____
_____
_____

Did your family celebrate with food? Explain.

_____
_____
_____

Did you ever get teased because of your weight? By whom?

_____
_____
_____

Has anyone told you that you need to lose weight? By whom?

_____
_____
_____

What feelings did you associate with food/overeating?

_____

_____

_____

Did you ever: Sneak/Hide food; were a picky eater; Binge eat; Throw-up; Starve yourself; worry about not having enough of your binge foods? Explain.

_____

_____

_____

What are your problem foods? What happens when you eat them?

_____

_____

_____

How do you feel after you eat your problem foods; binge or sneak eat?

_____

_____

_____

Do you have any co-morbidities? How long have you had them?

_____

_____

_____

What ways have you tried to lose weight? What were the outcomes?

_____

_____

_____

How do you feel about having bariatric surgery?

_____

_____

_____

How long have you researched bariatric surgery?

_____

_____

_____

Do you know anyone who had bariatric surgery? What was their results/thoughts about the outcome?

_____

_____

_____

What is your typical day like regarding meals, snacking or grazing?

_____

_____

_____

QUIZ: Do you have a healthy relationship with food? (Brabaw, 2019).

1. If you put too much food on your plate, you're more likely to...
A.   Put your fork down when you feel satisfied, even if there's still food on the plate.
B.   Put your fork down when you feel full.
C.   Keep eating even after you feel full.

2. You're out to dinner with friends and really want a piece of cheesecake for dessert. You...
A.   Get the cheesecake. It's okay to indulge once in a while.
B.   Only get the cheesecake if someone will split it, or if everyone else is getting dessert.
C.   Don't get the cheesecake but think about it all night.

3. Your best friend tells you all about a new diet that's supposed to make you lose weight quickly. You think...
A.   "I don't need a restrictive diet. I feel healthy eating the foods I like. "
B.   "I've tried those diets in the past, and they never work. Better stick to clean, healthy foods."
C.   "I've got to try this!"

4. On a typical day, you think about food...
A.   When you're hungry.
B.   When you're hungry or stressed.
C.   All the time.

5. You've heard about a new "superfood" that's supposed to be ridiculously good for you. You gave it a try, but don't like it. You...
A.   Will give it more than one chance but won't force yourself to eat it.
B.   Will never eat it again.
C.   Eat it at least once a week—and hate every moment of it.

6. All your friends are using calorie counter apps on their phones. They say you should try it, too. You think...
A.   "No, thanks. My body is better than any app at telling me when it's had enough food."
B.   "Maybe. I can't always tell if I'm full—a calorie counter might be able to help me determine when to stop."
C.   "Yes! I can't trust myself to eat only what my body needs."

7. It's a super-busy day at work, and you don't have time to grab breakfast. Your only option is the

bagels someone left in the break room. You...
A.   Grab a bagel—you're hungry and it's better than skipping breakfast.
B.   Get the bagel but eat only half even though you're still hungry.
C.   Skip breakfast. No way are you going to eat a bagel.

RESULTS

Mostly A's: You and food are best buds—in a good way.
No one has a perfect relationship with food. Chances are, you sometimes stress eat or overindulge. But if you eat mostly clean, healthy foods; can listen to your body and what it needs, and don't feel guilty when you have a treat, then congratulations: You have a healthy relationship with food.

Mostly B's: You and food have a love/hate relationship.
Most people fall into this middle area: Food isn't your whole life, but you make a good number of dietary decisions based on 1) what other people will think about what you're eating and 2) whether eating certain foods or not eating them will cause you to gain weight or help you lose it. Food isn't always on your

mind, and it doesn't get in the way of your quality of life, but it'd be lying to say you don't feel guilty whenever you eat too much or eat something you believe to be unhealthy, like a cupcake.

Mostly C's: You and food are mortal enemies. You think about food almost ALL the time. And those thoughts—which include what or when you'll eat next, how healthy your diet is, whether the food you eat will help you lose weight, and/or whether you've been "bad" for eating too much or a treat—interrupt your daily life; prevent you from enjoying food, meals, or social situations; and are possibly interfering with your health. If you fall into this group, you may need to get help. Disordered eating can take many forms, not just the anorexia and bulimia that most people are familiar with. For more information, visit the National Eating Disorders Association or consider seeing a therapist, psychologist, psychiatrist, or other trained specialists for help.

Stress Eating

"What hurts us is what heals us."

— Paulo Coelho

Studies show that women with high chronic stress levels tend to participate in emotional eating. Stress eating often begins with a *trigger*. Using food to combat stress can be a *mindless* activity. Without thinking, you just grab a snack or treat yourself to foods as a relief from your stress. Being aware of your responses to stress is one way to curb stress eating.

Stress is something everyone experiences in their personal and professional lives. But when stress is severe or prolonged (or both), it can impact your physical *and* mental health in major ways. Learn to recognize when you are feeling stress so you can make a *conscience* effort to not turn to food for comfort.

Managing Stress Eating

- **Practice Mindful Eating.**

    Know that your craving may be a result of a stressful event. Ask yourself, are you truly hungry? Wait a few minutes before eating.

- **Find Healthier Options.**

    If you still feel the need for a snack, consider a lower-calorie, lower-fat option than what you may have previously chosen.

- **Watch Portion Size.**

    Instead of taking the whole box with you, put a snack-size amount on a plate. Check the package to see what one serving size is and try to stick to that.

Do you eat over stress? What are your major stressors in your life?

_____

_____

_____

What are some of the things you have done to combat stress eating?

_____

_____

_____

What new healthy coping skills can you use instead of eat?

_____

_____

_____

My Mind

You are my friend,
And my enemy.
When I am up,
You mess it up.
When I am down
You tell me to reach
for food.
Why do I let you
Control my
thoughts
The way I do?
    — Anonymous

Chapter 2

Healing Your Mind

"If something stands between you and your success, move it. Never be denied."

— Dwayne "The Rock" Johnson

What some of the bariatric community has said:

1. Had to change the way I thought about myself and my body.
2. Re-learn who I am after weight loss.
3. Love and appreciate the body you are in.
4. I'd still see the fat person in the mirror.
5. That I wouldn't wake up loving myself.
6. Eat, move, act, and speak like you love yourself.
7. Food isn't comfort…it's fuel.
8. There's a difference between being full and satisfied.
9. Knowledge is my friend.

10. Treasure all the parts about you that makes you different and unique. You are beautiful.
11. Nothing's worked before, why should this be any different?
12. I feel hopeless.
13. I just want to eat.
14. Be patient.
15. My life was an absolute wreck, a nightmare. Never, ever to go back there again.
16. I still struggle with over-buying groceries.
17. I don't buy new clothes. Everything I have was from a thrift store except bras and undies.
18. How hard saying goodbye to my old self would be.
19. Love myself before.
20. Self-love is the beginning.
21. You're going to have good days and bad days.
22. Just remember you are going to be ok.
23. Keep your head up.
24. If you need to start over several times a day, do it 'til you feel better.

25. Love and appreciate the body you are in.
26. You are the greatest project you will ever work on.
27. Be kind to yourself.
28. Love yourself first and everything else falls into place.
29. An important part of mindful eating is to chew 30 times, take 30 minutes to eat and wait 30 minutes to drink after finishing eating.
30. I am trying to be mindful to eat all my protein, drink all my water and take all my vitamins daily.
31. Have great coping skills so that you don't turn to food again.
32. Have healthy replacements for turning to food.
33. Develop new hobbies.
34. One of my worst coping mechanisms has always been turning to food for comfort.
35. Replace binge eating with a non-food habit/hobby/coping mechanism.
36. It will be hard to let the clothes go.

37. Saying goodbye is hard.
38. Ready to say goodbye to my grandma looking clothes.
39. I got emotional every time I bagged up more to give away. I have some good friends that wear my old sizes, so I passed them along since we work in similar office-type setting.
40. I gave everything away. Made me feel better if it's a person in need. Women's shelters always could use job/interview appropriate clothing. Better than dropping them off at Goodwill.
41. Been there done that. I finally realized that the clothing pieces I felt very emotional about were my favorites! I had great memories of good times while wearing these clothes.
42. We spend a lot of time and money to find what we like and it's hard to let go. I finally was able to garage sale them with fill a bag price and when the person was leaving with said clothes I just had to say, "I hope you have as much fun in them as I did."

43. It was like me saying goodbye to some longtime friends. These clothes were my comfort zone. It's just time to invest in some "new feel-good clothing pieces."
44. I felt a lot more attachment than I though. Just remember to save before clothes.
45. The clothes are definitely an emotional crutch.
46. Stick to the plan…get rid of it! Just remember how you feel now compared to when you were the bigger size. New phase, new clothes, and new experiences.
47. Choose a few of your favorite pieces and have a memory blanket made out of them.
48. I had beautiful expensive clothes that I gave away. It's a new you. You may want a whole new look!
49. These clothes even at your heaviest made you feel a bit better about yourself. Now you don't need these clothes and a vacuum sometimes forms in our minds about I all.

50. It was great going shopping after losing weight. For the first time in my life, I was excited and happy to shop. The fact that I had to keep getting smaller and smaller sizes was amazing. I cried happy tears in the dressing room instead of sad tears.
51. I cried when I gave up my old clothes.
52. It's bittersweet. I've cried some mornings because I couldn't find anything that fit for work.
53. It's normal to grieve the "old" you which includes our clothes. I also thrift because I changed sizes so fast. But you will learn to love the new clothes too.
54. I had zero issues getting rid of anything. I wanted room for my new stuff!
55. Getting rid of my clothes was getting rid of part of me.
56. My heart and mind are strong.
57. I will own this new life!
58. I am making positive choices for a better life.

59. I love the new body I am getting.

60. I always remember where I came from.

61. Do…compliment yourself!

62. Uplift others on their journey.

63. If you believe you can or believe you can't…you are right.

Self-Esteem

"You don't become what you want, you become what you believe."

— Oprah

Self-esteem is how you value and respect yourself as a person. It is the opinion that you have of yourself inside and out. This impacts how you take care of yourself, emotionally, physically, and spiritually. Self-esteem is about your whole self, not just your body.

When you have *good* self-esteem, you value yourself, and you know that you deserve good care and respect—from yourself and from others. You can appreciate and celebrate your strengths and abilities, and you *don't* put yourself down if you make a mistake.

Good self-esteem means that you still feel like you're good enough *even* when you're dealing with difficult feelings or situations. Low self-esteem can cause you to turn to food to *deal* with feelings of inadequacy. "Beating yourself up" is a self-punishment because that's all you feel like you deserve. Low self-esteem can be a *common* element of eating disorders.

People with High Self-Esteem: (Ackerman, 2018)

- Appreciate themselves and other people.
- Enjoy growing as a person and finding fulfillment and meaning in their lives.
- Are able to dig deep within themselves and be creative.
- Make their own decisions and conform to what others tell them to be and do only when they agree.
- See the word in realistic terms, accepting other people the way they are while pushing them toward greater confidence and a more positive direction.

- Can easily concentrate on solving problems in their lives.
- Have loving and respectful relationships.
- Know what their values are and live their lives accordingly.
- Speak up and tell others their opinions, calmly and kindly, and share their wants and needs with others.
- Endeavor to make a constructive difference in other people's lives.

You Likely Have High Self-esteem if You: (Ackerman, 2018)

- Act assertively without experiencing any guilt and feel at ease communicating with others.
- Avoid dwelling on the past and focus on the present moment.
- Believe you are equal to everyone else, no better and no worse.
- Reject the attempts of others to manipulate you.

- Recognize and accept a wide range of feelings, both positive and negative, and share them within your healthy relationships.
- Enjoy a healthy balance of work, play, and relaxation.
- Accept challenges and take risks to grow and learn from your mistakes when you fail.
- Handle criticism without taking it personally, with the knowledge that you are learning and growing and that your worth is not dependent on the opinions of others.
- Value yourself and communicate well with others, without fear of expressing your likes, dislikes, and feelings.
- Value others and accept them as they are without trying to change them.

How do you feel about your body?

_____

_____

_____

How do you feel about your life?

_____

_____

_____

What are the things you feel like you have settled for in your life/relationships?

_____

_____

_____

Do you feel like you deserve better in your life/relationships? Explain.

_____

_____

_____

QUIZ: Self-esteem

Read each statement and circle your response.

Strongly Agree	Agree	Disagree	Strongly Disagree

Overall, I am satisfied with myself.

    3   2   1   0

At times, I think I am no good at all.

    0   1   2   3

I feel that I have many good qualities.

    3   2   1   0

I can do things as well as most other people.

    3   2   1   0

I feel I do not have much to be proud of.

    0   1   2   3

I certainly feel useless at times.

    0   1   2   3

I feel that I'm a person of worth, at least on an equal plane with others.

      3   2   1   0

I wish I could have more respect for myself.

      0   1   2   3

All in all, I tend to feel that I am a failure.

      0   1   2   3

I take a positive attitude toward myself.

      3   2   1   0

Add up the number of points in each response you circled. The higher the number, the higher your self-esteem.

Adapted from the Rosenberg Self-Esteem Scale excerpted from Canadian Mental Health Association, BC Division.

Shame

Shame is the lie someone told you about yourself. It is a soul eating emotion.

Shame is a *severe* form of embarrassment or humiliation. You can feel shame because of the way you look, something you've done, something done to you, how others have treated you, or how you think others perceive you. People might have even shamed you by saying, "You should be ashamed!" It can bring on feelings like self-loathing or hate towards yourself.

Bullying brings on another type of shame. It's the combination of what they tell or do to you, especially if it's in front of other people. Any type of abuse can cause you to feel shame because of what happened or how you have been made to feel like it's your fault. These types of past trauma can shape you into who you are today. But you *don't* have to stay there. Acknowledge what happened and *move on*. Put it behind you and forgive yourself and others.

Forgiveness is for *you* and not them. It's not to let anyone off the hook. But it's to kick them out of your head.

People who have had bariatric surgery *still* have to deal with shame. You may feel ashamed that you had to resort to surgery to lose weight. Or others may have pointed that out to you. You might have heard things like, "You took the easy way out," or "You cheated by having surgery to lose weight." Your self-perception of what you believe other people think of you could include being lazy or sloppy.

What things have made you feel shame?

_____

_____

_____

Who has shamed you? What have they done?

_____

_____

_____

What do you feel shame about today?

_____

_____

_____

What parts of your body make you feel shame?

_____

_____

_____

Body Image

"I definitely have body issues, but everybody does. When you come to the realization that everybody does that—even the people that I consider flawless—then you can start to live with the way you are."

— Taylor Swift

What do you think you look like? What do you *see* when you look in the mirror? How you feel about the way you look right now is your body image. Do your concerns focus on your height, weight, skin, hair, or the shape or size of a certain part of your body? It *begins* in your mind and contributes to your value and worth. Affecting your self-worth, it is both mental and emotional. A healthy body image is when you can *truly* accept and like the way you look.

Did you know that people who have been bullied are more likely to develop an eating disorder than others? Negative body image can come from bullying, and the bully doesn't always have to be the schoolyard's notorious character. You often see bullies attack the overweight, and then they turn to food to comfort themselves from the attacks.

Body image *directly* relates to self-esteem. If you don't like your body or parts of your body, it will be hard to like your entire body. It is possible to think about the unliked body part as being *separate* from the rest of your body.

Valuing yourself allows you to notice the good things about your body. Good body image, self-esteem, and mental health is about respecting yourself, thinking realistically, and taking action to deal with your problems in healthy ways. It is not about making yourself feel happy all the time.

Good body image and self-esteem positively impact mental health: (Canadian Mental Health Association, BC Division, 2015).

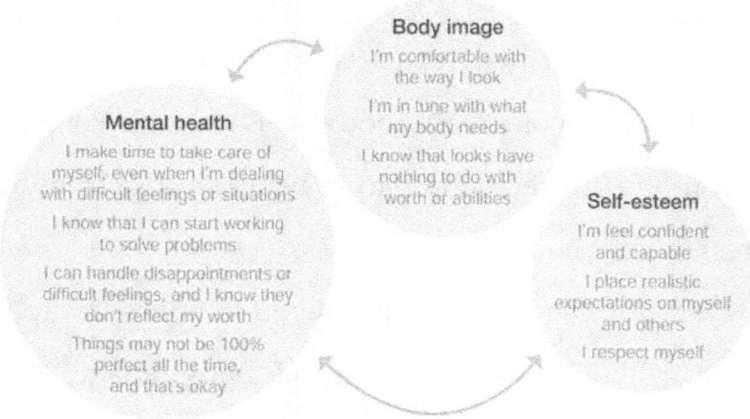

The problem with focusing on shortcomings or problems is that it becomes very *easy* to only see problems in other areas. Negative thinking and feelings can lead to *more* negative thinking. Poor body image can affect a person in many ways, including their academic performance, professional career, relationship satisfaction, and overall quality of life. If you have poor body image you may have a negative view of your body and obsess over how you look.

Signs of Poor Body Image:

- Focus and obsess over a minor flaw in your appearance
- View yourself as unattractive or ugly.
- Fear that other people can see your "deformity"
- You might be a perfectionist
- Avoid social activities
- Constantly groom and look at yourself in the mirror
- Constantly hides your perceived flaw with makeup or clothes
- Constantly compares your appearance to others
- Get excessive cosmetic procedures or surgery
- Asks others for reassurance ("Do I look fat in this?")
- Never satisfied with your appearance

Poor body image and self-esteem negatively impact mental health: (Canadian Mental Health Association, BC Division, 2015).

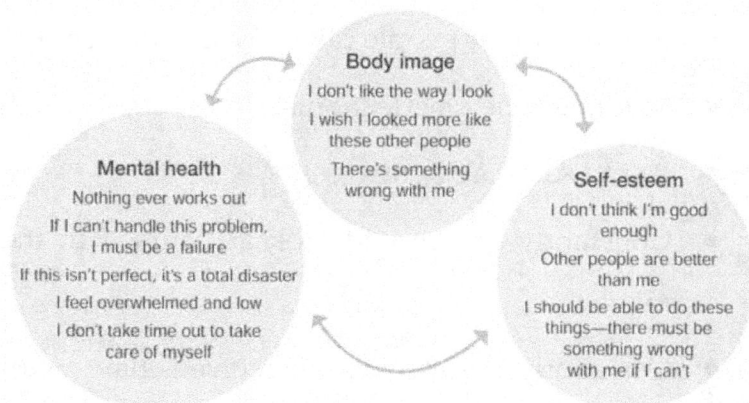

Tips to Having a Healthier Body Image:

- Respect your body
- Eat well and exercise
- Don't judge others by the way they look
- Dress to feel good about yourself
- Focus on a positive affirmation for the day
- Surround yourself with positive people

- Be aware of how you talk to others about your body
- Know that others have body image challenges too
- Write a list of all the positives about your body
- When negative thoughts come up, think about what you'd tell a friend
- Don't look at media that focuses on stereotypes
- Seek programs or information on positive coping skills

What do you see when you look at yourself in a mirror?

_____

_____

_____

What specific body parts you have problems with? Explain._____

_____

_____

Do you feel any of these feelings about your body? Shame, embarrassment, anxiety, low self-esteem, humiliation, self-consciousness, depression, isolation, lack of social interaction? Explain.

_____

_____

_____

Coping Skills

"I promise to stop analyzing every angle and every curve and every pound and every meal. I'm going to keep staying the path because it is a journey and as long as I'm always working towards my goals, one day I'll reach them."
— Carrie Underwood

Life after bariatric surgery will *forever* change you, both physically and mentally. Always remember the *why's* you chose to have the surgery. This will help you cope with the changes you will encounter. Having good coping skills to replace the ones you've always had is *especially* important to guarantee a lifetime of success. If you turned to food for comfort or support, now is the time that needs to change. Numbing the feelings will only be a *temporary* fix to your problems.

While turning to food to cope might help in the *short term*, the feelings of regret and guilt can lead to other negative emotions. You will need to find healthy replacements for food that you used as comfort and coping.

When you are *tempted* to turn to food, identify your feelings or emotions. Is there something going on in your life that you're trying to "stuff" your feelings over? Are you bored, stressed, anxious or just having a bad day? Are you triggered? It's important to stop and think first before you eat. Ask yourself questions to determine *why* you want to comfort with food.

Journaling daily is a good way to identify what you are going through and how you feel. Having a good support system can be a *great* way to deal with life. This could include your family, friends, other bariatric patients, or a support group.

Support groups meet online or in person. Don't be afraid to ask for help when you need help. That's what they are there for, to support you and each other.

If you feel like you *still* need help in giving up your old coping skills by turning to food, seek counseling. A therapist can guide you to identify your feelings, circumstances and help you to develop positive coping skills. Knowing *when* to seek counseling shows growth on your part because it's the *healthiest* people who know when they need help.

Ideas for Coping Skills other than Food:

- Get involved in activities you enjoy enhancing feelings of creativity and passion and boost your self-esteem
- Reach out and talk with friends
- Say positive affirmations
- Get a massage
- Walk or play with your dog
- Create a fun to-do list of activities with friends
- Learn a new skill, hobby, or take a class
- Make a gratitude list

Check all that you tried:

- ☐ Accept a challenge
- ☐ Ask for a hug
- ☐ Ask for help
- ☐ Be a tourist in your own city
- ☐ Belly breaths
- ☐ Blow bubbles
- ☐ Build something
- ☐ Call a friend
- ☐ Care for a pet
- ☐ Change a negative thought into a positive one
- ☐ Clean the house
- ☐ Close your eyes and relax
- ☐ Coloring
- ☐ Cook a meal
- ☐ Count to 10 or 100
- ☐ Create jewelry
- ☐ Cry
- ☐ Dance
- ☐ Do a crossword puzzle

- ☐ Do a positive activity
- ☐ Do a puzzle
- ☐ Do a word search
- ☐ Doodle on paper
- ☐ Donate clothes
- ☐ Do something creative
- ☐ Do yoga
- ☐ Draw a comic
- ☐ Draw or paint
- ☐ Drink enough water
- ☐ Drink tea
- ☐ Eat a healthy snack
- ☐ Enjoy nature
- ☐ Exercise
- ☐ Explore somewhere new
- ☐ Face your problems
- ☐ Feel your feelings
- ☐ Find humor
- ☐ Flip through a magazine
- ☐ Get enough sleep
- ☐ Get some sunshine

- ☐ Go for a bike ride
- ☐ Go for a walk
- ☐ Go out for coffee
- ☐ Go rock climbing
- ☐ Go stargazing
- ☐ Go swimming
- ☐ Go to a concert
- ☐ Go to a play
- ☐ Go to the beach
- ☐ Go to the library
- ☐ Grounding exercises
- ☐ Hang out with friends
- ☐ Have a picnic
- ☐ Hike on a nature trail
- ☐ Hug a loved one or pillow
- ☐ Ignore negative people
- ☐ Kindness to yourself or others
- ☐ Knit
- ☐ Laugh out loud
- ☐ Learn something new on YouTube
- ☐ Limit caffeine

- ☐ Listen to the radio or podcast
- ☐ List your positive qualities
- ☐ List your strengths
- ☐ Look at old pictures
- ☐ Make a gratitude list
- ☐ Make origami
- ☐ Meditate
- ☐ Meet someone new
- ☐ Open up to friends or family
- ☐ Paint your nails
- ☐ Plant some seeds
- ☐ Play a board game or card game
- ☐ Play a musical instrument
- ☐ Play a sport
- ☐ Play a video game
- ☐ Play cards
- ☐ Play with a child
- ☐ Play with a pet
- ☐ Play with clay
- ☐ Play with fidget toys
- ☐ Practice deep/slow breathing

- ☐ Practice mindfulness
- ☐ Pray
- ☐ Punch a pillow or your bed
- ☐ Question negative thoughts
- ☐ Read a book
- ☐ Read a joke book
- ☐ Read a newspaper
- ☐ Read inspirational quotes
- ☐ Rearrange your furniture
- ☐ Research an unfamiliar topic online
- ☐ Rip paper into pieces
- ☐ Run, walk or jog
- ☐ Say "I can do this"
- ☐ Say something kind
- ☐ Schedule time for yourself
- ☐ Scream into a pillow
- ☐ Search for new music to listen to
- ☐ Set a new goal
- ☐ Shop at the thrift store
- ☐ Sing
- ☐ Sit in nature

- ☐ Smile
- ☐ Squeeze a stress ball
- ☐ Spend time with family
- ☐ Stand up and stretch
- ☐ Start a blog
- ☐ Surf the web
- ☐ Talk to a therapist
- ☐ Talk to your pet
- ☐ Take a bubble bath
- ☐ Take a break
- ☐ Take a nap
- ☐ Take a shower
- ☐ Take pictures
- ☐ Take some alone time
- ☐ Take the dog for a walk
- ☐ Take photos
- ☐ Try a new food or recipe
- ☐ Try a new restaurant
- ☐ Unplug from phone/social media
- ☐ Use aromatherapy
- ☐ Use positive affirmations

- ☐ Use positive self-talk
- ☐ Visit a friend
- ☐ Visit a museum
- ☐ Visit neighbors
- ☐ Visit a park
- ☐ Visit a tourist attraction
- ☐ Visualize a peaceful place
- ☐ Visualize your favorite place
- ☐ Volunteer
- ☐ Watch a movie or TV show
- ☐ Watch the sunrise or sunset
- ☐ Work in the garden
- ☐ Write a book
- ☐ Write a letter
- ☐ Write a list
- ☐ Write a poem
- ☐ Write a short story
- ☐ Write in a journal
- ☐ Write your own song

ADD YOUR OWN:

1.

2.

3.

4.

5.

Letting Go

"Let go of the past."

— Robert Greene

Letting go of the *old* you is part of the process towards the *newer* healthier you. This task will be difficult and challenging. But it is necessary to do to move forward in your new life. There are positive benefits just waiting for you.

Remembering where you came from is one important part of letting go. This can be a *great* motivator to continue with your new bariatric life. Your old life has probably been with you longer than this new journey and is familiar. Yet it can be a painful part of your life. Embrace it. Love it. Accept it. Then, *let it go!*

Acceptance brings freedom and peace. It is not saying that you *like* it, but rather "it is what it is." Acceptance will bring you peace to look at where you came from and *not* beat yourself up over it. You did the best that you could with what you had to do it with. You got through it. You survived. Now you have a do-over, a *new* chance at a better healthier life.

One of the most powerful things you can do is write yourself a letter. Fully express how you feel about having to let the old you go. Write about your life and how you survived and coped. Talk about how this new life is a *blessing* and you're not leaving the old you behind. You are bettering yourself and bringing your old self along for the ride. Keep this letter and read it periodically. Letting go of the old you is *not* saying goodbye. It's saying, "Please come along with me on this new adventure."

Letting go of the bigger clothes is also part of the process towards your new healthier life. This can also be *quite* a challenge. The clothes have been with you probably for a long time. They are your friends, comfort, and were there for you in the hard times of your life. Keep an outfit at your highest weight. You can use this as a motivational tool to see how far you've come. Some people use their old clothes and make a quilt out of them.

At some point you will have to part ways with your bigger clothes and get some new ones. Look at this as an *exciting* journey! Shop in your closet. If you are like most people, you have many sizes just hanging in your closet. Donate your clothes or gift to others that may need it. Bring to shelter's or sell them. There are ways to say goodbye to your bigger clothes and realize you are *blessing* others just as they were once blessing you.

Don't buy a lot of new clothes as you will change sizes rapidly. Thrift shop or just buy a few pieces of clothes. Get a goal outfit and hang it up. Look at it often and picture yourself in that outfit. When you can wear it, buy yourself another *smaller* goal outfit. Smaller tighter clothes will become more comfortable that the bigger loose ones. Trust the journey, you will be *excited* to get smaller clothes!

How do you feel about letting go of the old you?

_____

_____

_____

What is the hardest part of letting go?

_____

_____

_____

What is something positive about letting go of the old you?

_____

_____

_____

How do you feel about letting go of the bigger clothes?

_____

_____

_____

What is the hardest part of letting the clothes go?

_____

_____

_____

What is something positive about letting go of the bigger clothes?

_____

_____

_____

Love Thyself

"He is a <u>wise</u> man who does not grieve for the things which he has not, but rejoices for those which he has."
— Epictetus

Love yourself *first*. When it's all said and done you are the best person to take care of you! You are your best advocate. If you're not happy, it can affect everyone around you. Plus, loving yourself will make you happier overall. You *deserve* that respect!

Every day make it your goal to work on yourself. Schedule yourself in your daily life. Only *you* can change you. Check in with yourself every day and see how you feel and if there are things you can work on. Loving yourself has *nothing* to do with if you're happy with your life circumstances. If you can make changes, then do it. Set small attainable goals and go for it!

Know that your past *can* affect how much you love yourself. If you've had trauma or painful events, it can affect how you feel about yourself. Acknowledge your experiences and pain and *still* love yourself. Don't let it interfere with how you feel about yourself.

If there were some things you did wrong or made bad choices, forgive *yourself*. Examine if you need to apologize to others for actions you did wrong. This is for *you*, so you can forgive yourself. If you feel like you can't move on from your past or feel stuck there, seek counseling.

Acceptance is *freedom* from any negative thoughts of things that may have happened. Accept where you are, exactly as you are. Acceptance is not agreeing or liking a situation. It is saying, "It is what it is." This will give you peace of mind. It's not to let anyone off the hook for their actions or behaviors. It's for *you… your peace of mind.*

I accept these people:

_____

_____

_____

I accept these things they have done to me:

_____

_____

_____

I accept these life situations I have no control over:

_____

_____

_____

What changes can I make to change my life situations?

_____

_____

_____

Positive Affirmations

If I can change my mind, I can change anything.

Your mind is powerful. What you tell it, will *grow*. When you fill it up with positive thoughts, your life will begin to change in a *positive* way. Telling yourself positive messages every day is such a positive part of success. Telling yourself positive affirmations regularly helps to build confidence, self-esteem, and self-worth.

Eliminate negative thinking by turning your negative thoughts into positive thoughts. Every time you think something negative, stop, think, and change the thought into a positive one.

Example: I just can't do this program right.

Change: For today, I will do the best that I can do.

Example: I just want to eat what I could eat before.

Change: Good food nourishes my body and is good for me.

Pick a positive affirmation that you can relate to. Believe in the power of saying it every day. You can also pick one that you want to *start* believing about yourself. In time, you will come to believe it to be true. Look at yourself and areas that need changing. Then add your own positive affirmation to the list below.

Check all that you say. Keep adding to your list of positive affirmations:

- ☐ Being active is great for my body
- ☐ Every day brings me one step closer to my goal
- ☐ Every day I recognize my progress
- ☐ Everything I eat heals my body
- ☐ Exercise has become an important part of my routine
- ☐ I accept and acknowledge my body shape and the beauty it holds

- ☐ I accept my body right where I am
- ☐ I accept myself for who I am and where I am
- ☐ I allow love into my heart
- ☐ I allow myself to make choices for what's best for me
- ☐ I am always kind and loving to my body
- ☐ I am a work of art
- ☐ I am determined to be successful I am determined to reach my goals
- ☐ I am eating foods that contribute to my wellness
- ☐ I am full of confidence and determination
- ☐ I am happily achieving my weight loss goals
- ☐ I am healthy and strong
- ☐ I am improving my lifestyle by losing weight
- ☐ I am losing weight because I want to
- ☐ I am making the right choices with my health
- ☐ I am not addicted to food
- ☐ I am succeeding at this new lifestyle
- ☐ I am taking small realistic steps towards success
- ☐ I am thankful for my body

- ☐ I believe in my awesomeness!
- ☐ I believe in myself and recognize my greatness
- ☐ I can achieve anything I want
- ☐ I can now see myself at my ideal weight
- ☐ I choose to eat food that's beneficial for my body
- ☐ I crave nutritious food
- ☐ I create my future
- ☐ I don't care how others feel about my body
- ☐ I don't compare myself to others
- ☐ I don't eat out of emotions
- ☐ I drink enough water to stay hydrated
- ☐ I eat slowly and chew well to digest properly
- ☐ I eliminate negative thoughts regarding the process
- ☐ I enjoy creating healthy habits that I will continue throughout my life
- ☐ I enjoy drinking water and staying hydrated
- ☐ I enjoy eating healthy food
- ☐ I feel good just being me
- ☐ I feel great in my skin

- [ ] I feel great about myself
- [ ] I have everything I need to reach my goals
- [ ] I have healthy attainable goals
- [ ] I have hope about my future
- [ ] I have fulfillment, happiness, and contentment in my life as I am now
- [ ] I have the support of my friends and family
- [ ] I focus on my own journey
- [ ] I know discipline and persistence are necessary for losing weight
- [ ] I know that losing weight takes time
- [ ] I let go of any guilt I hold around unhealthy food choices
- [ ] I let go of stress related to losing weight
- [ ] I let go of the things that triggers my eating
- [ ] I let go of unhealthy patterns of behavior around food
- [ ] I like taking care of my body and mind
- [ ] I like what I see in the mirror
- [ ] I love me
- [ ] I love how I feel after exercising

- ☐ I love that my body is becoming stronger
- ☐ I love to spend time in nature
- ☐ I'm proud of my successful progress
- ☐ I only eat when I feel hungry
- ☐ I recognize my inside and outside beauty
- ☐ I take time to think before I give into cravings
- ☐ It's all about me!
- ☐ I truly love myself for who I am
- ☐ I've got this!
- ☐ I will be the person I want in my life
- ☐ I will continue eating healthy even after I reach my goal
- ☐ I will donate my big clothes with love
- ☐ I will make time for me
- ☐ I will not be impulsive
- ☐ I will put myself as a priority
- ☐ I woke up winning
- ☐ Losing weight is worth the struggle
- ☐ My body craves healthy foods
- ☐ My body needs healthy food

- ☐ My body looks amazing
- ☐ My energy levels increase every time I eat healthy
- ☐ My health is my priority
- ☐ The food choices I make are consistent with my ultimate goal in losing weight and being healthy
- ☐ The food I choose to eat nourishes my body
- ☐ The most important things are my physical and mental health
- ☐ The number on the scale doesn't define who I am or my progress
- ☐ Today I don't need to be perfect
- ☐ When I eat healthy food, I feel energized
- ☐ When I look in the mirror, I see a healthy beautiful person

ADD YOUR OWN:

1.

2.

3.

4.

5.

Mindfulness

"Do every act of your life as though it was the very last act of your life."

— Marcus Aurelius

Mindfulness is the basic human ability to be fully present in the moment. You are intensely aware of what you're sensing and feeling, where you are and what you're doing. It's a state of not being overwhelmed or reactive to what's going on around you.

If practiced daily, mindfulness will be more readily available to you, although it is something everyone naturally possesses. Whenever you bring awareness to what you're directly experiencing through your senses, or to your state of mind through your thoughts and emotions, you're being mindful.

The goal of mindfulness is to wake up the inner workings of your mental, emotional, and physical state. Make it your goal to practice mindfulness *every* day for six months and you might find that mindfulness becomes effortless. You will be able to reconnect with and nurture yourself. Simple mindfulness exercises can be practiced anywhere and anytime. Research shows that engaging your senses outdoors is especially beneficial.

Simple Ways to Practice Mindfulness:

- **Pay Attention.** It's hard to slow down and notice things in a busy world. Try to take the time to experience your environment with all your senses — touch, sound, sight, smell, and taste. For example, when you eat a favorite food, take the time to smell, taste and truly enjoy it.
- **Live in the Moment.** Try to intentionally bring an open, accepting, and discerning attention to everything you do. Find joy in simple pleasures.
- **Accept Yourself.** Treat yourself the way you would treat a good friend.

- **Focus on your Breathing.** When you have negative thoughts, try to sit down, take a deep breath, and close your eyes. Focus on your breath as it moves in and out of your body. Sitting and breathing for even just a minute can help.

Mindful Eating

Distracted eating is when you are doing something else while you eat – such as watching TV, texting, surfing the web, driving, or talking on the phone. Times like these prevent you from being fully aware of how much you are eating, tastes of food and from entirely enjoying your food.

Since your mind is somewhere else, it can be *easy* to overeat or not be satisfied although you're no longer hungry. Being mindful while eating can help you focus on your food and the pleasure of your meal when you remove all outside distractions. Enjoy *all* your senses during the eating process, including what the food looks, smells, and tastes like, and even the experience of the texture of the food.

Mindful Meditation

Mindful meditation involves various types of meditation such as breathing methods, guided imagery, and other practices to relax the body and mind and help reduce stress. When you spend too much time planning, problem-solving, daydreaming, or thinking negative or random thoughts, it can be draining. You will more than likely experience stress, anxiety, and symptoms of depression. Practicing mindfulness exercises will help you direct your attention away from this kind of thinking and engage in the world around you.

Meditation allows you to go into your mind and sense what is around you. This includes tapping into *all* your senses. It can help you experience thoughts and emotions with greater balance and acceptance. Benefits of meditation include reducing stress, anxiety, pain, depression, insomnia, and high blood pressure. Also, meditation has been shown to *improve* attention, decrease job burnout, improve sleep, and improve diabetes control. You'll need to set aside time when you can be in a quiet place without distractions or interruptions to do the meditations.

Structured Mindfulness Exercises Include:

- **Body Scan Meditation.** Lie on your back with your legs extended and arms at your sides, palms facing up. Focus your attention slowly and deliberately on each part of your body, in order, from toe to head or head to toe. Be aware of any sensations, emotions or thoughts associated with each part of your body.
- **Sitting Meditation.** Sit comfortably with your back straight, feet flat on the floor and hands in your lap. Breathing through your nose, focus on your breath moving in and out of your body. If physical sensations or thoughts interrupt your meditation, note the experience, and then return your focus to your breath.

- **Walking Meditation.** Find a quiet place 10 to 20 feet in length and begin to walk slowly. Focus on the experience of walking, being aware of the sensations of standing and the subtle movements that keep your balance. When you reach the end of your path, turn, and continue walking, maintaining awareness of your sensations.
- **Grounding Meditation.** The body awareness technique will bring you into the here-and-now by directing your focus to sensations in the body. Pay special attention to the physical sensations created by each step.
    1. Take 5 long, deep breaths through your nose, and exhale through puckered lips.
    2. Place both feet flat on the floor. Wiggle your toes. Curl and uncurl your toes several times. Spend a moment noticing the sensations in your feet.
    3. Stomp your feet on the ground several times. Pay attention to the sensations in your feet and legs as you contact the ground.

4. Clench your hands into fists, then release the tension. Repeat this 10 times.
5. Press your palms together. Press them harder and hold this pose for 15 seconds. Pay attention to the feeling of tension in your hands and arms.
6. Rub your palms together briskly. Notice and sound and the feeling of warmth.
7. Reach your hands over your head like you're trying to reach the sky. Stretch like this for 5 seconds. Bring your arms down and let them relax at your sides.
8. Take 5 more deep breaths and notice the feeling of calm in your body.

Goodbye Friend

You used to be my friend, my comfort, my joy.
The friend who only gave me temporary fulfillment.
Then turned on me.
You made me unhealthy with diseases and excess weight.
But now I must tell you goodbye.
I no longer need you to exist.
I have a better and healthier way of life.
But I will miss you friend.

— Anonymous

Chapter 3

Social Changes

"If you gauge your life on what other people think, you're going to be in a constant state of panic trying to please everyone. People should just concentrate on their own lives and their own health and their own happiness, and whatever that looks like for you, be happy with it."

— Kelly Clarkson

What some of the bariatric community has said:

1. I won't fit in some social situations anymore.
2. People will look and treat me different now that I've lost weight.
3. Divorce can happen.
4. I am grateful for my husband who loved me over the years of weight gain and never told me an unkind word.
5. Jealousy is real.
6. Relationships change.
7. Friends who were supportive are not now.

8. Not everyone will be happy about my progress.
9. Not everyone will understand you. But the ones that do will never forget you.
10. Not everyone will understand your journey. That's fine. It's not their journey to make sense of. It's yours.
11. It's terrible that some people will treat you nicer now that you are thinner.
12. Be careful who you tell.
13. If your husband doesn't want you to leave him, he should make sure he acts correctly following your surgery.
14. Have a support system in place.
15. Go to support group meetings.
16. Don't isolate, seek support.
17. Talk to more people who had bariatric surgery.
18. Join as many Facebook bariatric support groups as you can.
19. Support is to build each other up.
20. People smile at me now since I've lost weight. That makes me a little sad for the person I was

Relationships

"When someone shows you who they are, believe them the first time."

— Maya Angelou

Relationships *will* change after you have bariatric surgery. They may even start to change *when* you make the decision to have the surgery. You will have those people who were very supportive of you getting the surgery, but not so happy with your progress when you lose weight. They may decide for you when you have lost enough weight, tell you negative comments, or sabotage you.

Spouses or significant others may become jealous, claim you've changed too much, become insecure or question if you're cheating. If there is *already* weakness in the relationship, you will have more problems now. Underlying issues in the relationship will pop up. They might resent you and your progress. Watch out for sabotage! When they are your caregiver, they may get upset when you gain some independence and not rely on them as much. Or they may not like the added attention you are being given, especially of the opposite sex. They may pay more attention to you. Stand up for yourself and let them know what is and what is not acceptable to you.

People report getting a divorce or a breakup and have blamed bariatric surgery. Don't be one of them. Keep open communication with your spouse or significant other along the way. Keeping them in the loop of your changes will make them feel a part of your journey. Ask their opinions and it will make them feel important in your life. Consider couples counseling before and after surgery to address any problems *already* in the relationship or as new ones come up.

Friendships can also change. If you were always the "fat friend" and now you're *not*, relationship dynamics will change. There could be some jealously involved. If you lose friends because you have chosen to have a healthier life, then so be it. Were they really that good of friends anyway if they aren't still supportive?

The opposite can be true as well. People can treat you *nicer* now that you're thinner. Overweight people have reported being treated as if they are "invisible," even passed up for jobs, or overlooked for promotions. Feelings of sadness for the person you were, can arise.

Deciding who to tell you are having bariatric surgery should be a *careful* decision. Different people have their own opinions about bariatric surgery and may try to impose these opinions on you. Know that these people who know about your surgery may watch what you're eating or constantly talk to you about your progress. Remember, once you tell someone, you cannot *un*-tell them.

Social situations will change too. You will no longer be able to socialize and participate in eating foods that you use to enjoy before surgery. Always be *prepared* for any social event by either bringing a dish of something you can eat or stashing a snack in your purse or car. People who don't know about your surgery may notice that you aren't eating the way you did before and may even pressure you into "trying" something. Be strong! You can do this!!

What relationships are you worried about? Who? Why?

1.

2.

3.

4.

5.

Boundaries

"I've worked too hard and too long to let anything stand in the way of my goals."

— Mia Hamm

Setting and implementing personal boundaries is where the recognition of your personal space begins and other people's end. It is one of the most *empowering* actions you can do for yourself. However, it can be challenging for you if you've never spoken up for yourself or stated your needs. But you *must* love yourself enough to not let anyone use or abuse you. *You* are in control of your life. The more you value yourself, the healthier your boundaries will be.

Setting boundaries involves anything that affects you, your body, or your emotions. Boundaries can improve your overall health and well-being by allowing you to not lose yourself or give too much. When you *lack* boundaries, you can feel emotionally exhausted.

Friendships are overall essential to your health and happiness but without boundaries, they can disrupt your well-being. Once you set boundaries, you *need* to keep them. Let people clearly know how you want and expect to be treated. Along with that it is important for you to respect other's boundaries.

Not everyone will be happy with your boundaries. If they get angry, you need to re-evaluate whether they are toxic or if they are the ones you need boundaries with. Learn the art of disappointing and upsetting others, hurting feelings, and live with the reality that not all people will like you even though it won't be easy. Standing up for yourself leads to living an authentic and meaningful life that reflects your deepest desires, values, and needs.

You *must* decide what is best for you. This plays an important role is setting your boundaries and will affect your mental, emotional, and physical well-being. Consider what you will and will not accept. Setting boundaries will lead to self-fulfillment and contentment.

Personal Boundary Tips:

- **Define your Limits**

  Determining your limits helps you set boundaries. Consider how the boundary will affect you. Take your time in identifying your limits. You can reflect on past experiences that may have led to negative feelings or situations. Focus on what you want to accomplish. Prioritize you own personal values.

- **Evaluate your Relationships**

  Each relationship will vary with what boundaries you set. Think about each one separately and evaluate what needs to change in that relationship. If there is an unbalance, consider what type of boundary will help. Depending on the role you play in the relationship will dictate what boundary you need to set.

- **Communicate Clearly and be Assertive**

  The best way to set boundaries is to communicate them clearly to the other person. Be persistent in letting them know your limits. Ask that they respect your wishes.

- **Uphold your Boundaries**

  When someone crosses your boundary, you must be firm and uphold your boundary. If not, they will continue to disrespect your request. Explain to them why it is important for them to respect your wishes. Don't feel bad for upholding your boundary. Those that care about you will respect your decision.

What boundaries do you want to set and with whom?

1.

2.

3.

4.

5.

How do you plan to discuss your boundaries with these people?

_____

_____

_____

How will you handle those that disregard your boundaries?

_____

_____

_____

Support

"Ask for help. Not because you are weak. But because you want to remain strong."

— Les Brown

Bariatric surgery is a *lifetime* commitment. It is vital to have a support system in place for this journey. You should get a support system in place *before* you have the actual surgery. The first few days after the surgery will be the hardest time and you will need help. Make sure you have someone at the hospital with you. As you progress in your eating, having someone who can help you at home is helpful.

Talk to others who have had the surgery and ask many questions. Just remember that all people's journeys are *different*. You may or may not experience the same things as them. Join as many Facebook bariatric support groups as you can. Some are specific to the type of surgery you will have. You'll learn your favorite groups and develop many friendships and support. Even your doctor's office may have their own support group.

Check your phone for available apps that will track your progress. Ask others which ones are better and what they do. Especially in the beginning, it will be crucial to track your intake. When you stall you can evaluate if it's something you ate or just a normal part of your progress. Who you pick as your support system is essential. Pick these family members and friends wisely who will be there with you through thick and thin.

A support system can be a spouse/partner, parents, siblings, children, friends, teachers, or coaches. Even *better* would be to add to your support system someone who has had the surgery and has been successful with it. Rely upon your bariatric team as support too. Your bariatric team includes your dietician, doctor, nurses, therapist, and any other healthcare professionals that you need.

YOUR SUPPORT SYSTEM:

1.

2.

3.

4.

5.

Don't wait for someone

to bring you

flowers.

Plant your own garden

and decorate

your own soul

— luther burbank

Chapter 4

Mental Health Issues

"Although the world is full of suffering, it is full also of the overcoming of it."

— Helen Keller

What some of the bariatric community has said:

1. I have binged and purged for years.
2. I am afraid to eat.
3. Can I develop an eating disorder after surgery?
4. Make sure you have the right support and new coping skills to deal with underlying mental illness, food addiction, or trauma.
5. Body dysmorphia is a real mental health diagnosis.
6. How I still see myself at my top weight.
7. Re-learn who I am after weight loss.

8. Body dysmorphia is real. Sometimes when you see your thinner self you see the old body in the mirror.
9. Sometimes I don't recognize myself when I see my reflection in a building window.
10. Seek therapy for transferring addictions.
11. Food addiction is real.
12. I changed addictions.
13. My spending is out of control.
14. I chose sober because I wanted a better life. I stay sober because I got one.
15. Unfortunately, we're food addicts and have made bad habits before our surgery.
16. I recognized that I needed help and sought out counseling.
17. I left my manipulative husband and finally healing and improving.
18. It's like living in hell every day of my life.
19. My therapist has been my saving grace.
20. It's easier to manage before surgery.

21. It's the constant digs people make at me that make me want to turn to food.
22. People saying "I think you've lost enough, you're going to look sick."
23. A huge trigger is when there is a hurricane in the Gulf of Mexico.
24. Pat downs at the airport because I don't look like my picture anymore.
25. I can't go to movies and smell popcorn.
26. It's a trigger for me to focus on everything I put in my mouth.
27. Men who don't take No, trigger me.
28. I can't even walk into a bakery. Hell, even wedding receptions trigger me.
29. Festival food makes me go crazy.
30. Seeing adults with both parents is a huge trigger for me.
31. Every day I feel soooooo big still.
32. When I look at myself in the mirror, I see the most imperfections.

Anxiety

"No amount of anxiety can change the future."

— Karen Salmansohn

Life is full of ups and downs. There are many bumps in the road. Anxiety and stress are a normal part of life. You may have anxiety leading up to your bariatric surgery. This is normal. There are many unknowns about surgery and the outcomes. Learning healthy coping skills to deal with anxiety and stress will help you to live a happy life.

When anxiety consumes you, impairs your daily life and are difficult to control, you may have an anxiety disorder. Anxiety disorders are often characterized by excessive worry, fear, panic attacks, restlessness, muscle tension, flashbacks, nightmares, obsessions, and compulsions. Sometimes when your anxiety gets out of control you can go into a panic attack. Panic attacks feel like someone is sitting on your chest, have short breaths, increased heartrate, racing thoughts, and shakiness. It is hard to breathe and calm down. Panic attacks occur rapidly and is a buildup of anxiety. If you think you might have an anxiety disorder, seek a therapist or psychiatrist to diagnose you.

Common Anxiety Signs and Symptoms Include: (Mayoclinic, 2023)

- Feeling nervous, restless or tense
- Having a sense of impending danger, panic or doom
- Having an increased heart rate
- Breathing rapidly (hyperventilation)
- Sweating
- Trembling
- Feeling weak or tired
- Trouble concentrating or thinking about anything other than the present worry
- Having trouble sleeping
- Experiencing gastrointestinal (GI) problems

- Having difficulty controlling worry
- Having the urge to avoid things that trigger anxiety

What things in your daily life cause you anxiety?

_____

_____

_____

Have you ever had a panic attack? Explain.

_____

_____

_____

What was going on to cause your panic attack?

_____

_____

_____

What symptoms did you have when you had a panic attack?

_____

_____

_____

Depression

Life is not the way it is supposed to be...it is the way it is...the way we cope with it, is what makes the difference.

Depression feels like you are scared, sad, and tired all at the same time. You can have a fear of failure but feel stuck and unmotivated to do anything. You may want friends but have no desire to socialize. You may feel like you want to be alone but not want to be lonely. There are things in your life that need to be done, but you can't get started or get out of bed.

Ever have those days where you just want to crawl in bed and cover your head with the covers? *Any* overwhelming feeling consumes you. All of these feelings can happen at once and then you just feel numb.

Although depression can occur once in your life it is more common to have reoccurring episodes. During these episodes, symptoms occur most of the day, nearly every day. It causes severe symptoms that affect how you feel, think, and handle daily activities, such as sleeping, eating, or working. If you think you might have depression, seek a therapist or psychiatrist to diagnose you.

Symptoms of Depression: (Mayoclinic, 2023)

- Feelings of sadness, tearfulness, emptiness, or hopelessness
- Angry outbursts, irritability or frustration, even over small matters
- Loss of interest or pleasure in most or all normal activities, such as sex, hobbies or sports
- Sleep disturbances, including insomnia or sleeping too much
- Tiredness and lack of energy, so even small tasks take extra effort
- Reduced appetite and weight loss or increased cravings for food and weight gain
- Anxiety, agitation, or restlessness
- Slowed thinking, speaking or body movements

- Feelings of worthlessness or guilt, fixating on past failures or self-blame
- Trouble thinking, concentrating, making decisions and remembering things
- Frequent or recurrent thoughts of death, suicidal thoughts, suicide attempts or suicide
- Unexplained physical problems, such as back pain or headaches

Depression can also Involve Other Changes in Mood or Behavior that Include: (Ninh, 2023)

- Increased anger or irritability
- Feeling restless or on edge
- Becoming withdrawn, negative, or detached
- Increased engagement in high-risk activities
- Greater impulsivity
- Increased use of alcohol or drugs
- Isolating from family and friends
- Inability to meet the responsibilities of work and family or ignoring other important roles

- Problems with sexual desire and performance

What is going on in your life to make you feel depressed?

_____

_____

_____

What symptoms do you have to make you think you have depression?

_____

_____

_____

What have you done to combat depression?

_____

_____

_____

Eating Disorders

"If you want to fly, you've got to give up the stuff that weighs you down."

— Toni Morrison

Has your eating gotten so bad that you can't control it? Do you focus too much on food, body shape, or weight. Do you think you might have an eating disorder? Anyone can develop an eating disorder. Eating disorders are *not* just about food. In addition, they involve the mind.

The most common eating disorders are anorexia nervosa, bulimia nervosa, and binge-eating disorder. Anorexia nervosa is when you severely restrict your intake of food. Bulimia nervosa is when you binge eat and then purge through vomiting or overexercising. Binge-eating disorder is when you binge eat.

If you aren't sure if you have an eating disorder, then see a mental health professional that can assess and diagnose you. If you do have an eating disorder know that the bariatric life will be more difficult for you. Just because you had your body surgically changed doesn't mean that your *mind* will be changed. You will still have to face the demons that you dealt with before.

To have complete success, seek therapy and work out all the reasons you have an eating disorder. It is imperative for success to work out all the emotional and mental issues you may have. Before your bariatric surgery is the best time to work on your issues. You might also want to continue working on it after surgery.

Mental and Behavioral Signs may Include: (Seitz, 2022)

- dramatic weight loss
- concern about eating in public
- preoccupation with weight, food, calories, fat grams, or dieting

- complaints of constipation, cold intolerance, abdominal pain, lethargy, or excess energy
- excuses to avoid mealtime
- intense fear of weight gain or being "fat"
- dressing in layers to hide weight loss or stay warm
- severely limiting and restricting the amount and types of food consumed
- refusing to eat certain foods
- denying feeling hungry
- expressing a need to "burn off" calories
- repeatedly weighing oneself
- patterns of binge eating and purging
- developing rituals around food
- excessively exercising
- cooking meals for others without eating
- missing menstrual periods (in people who would typically menstruate)

Physical Signs may Include: (Seitz, 2022)

- stomach cramps and other gastrointestinal symptoms
- difficulty concentrating
- atypical lab test results (anemia, low thyroid levels, low hormone levels, low potassium, low blood cell counts, slow heart rate)
- dizziness
- fainting
- feeling cold all the time
- sleep irregularities
- menstrual irregularities
- calluses across the tops of the finger joints (a sign of inducing vomiting)
- dry skin
- dry, thin nails
- thinning hair
- muscle weakness
- poor wound healing
- poor immune system function

How are you preoccupied with food?

_____

_____

_____

What ways have you tried to control your eating and weight?

_____

_____

_____

Do you think you have an eating disorder? Why or why not?

_____

_____

_____

Body Dysmorphia

"Perfectionism is a self-destructive and addictive belief system that fuels this primary thought: If I look perfect, and do everything perfectly, I can avoid or minimize the painful feelings of shame, judgment, and blame."

— Brené Brown

Who do you see when you look in the mirror? Do you still see the overweight person? Do you notice every bump, lump, and wrinkle? Do these thoughts consume you and affect your thoughts and actions? Body dysmorphia disorder (BDD) can overwhelm and overtake your mind. BDD can impact your quality of life and how you feel about yourself.

When you have BDD you believe that you are "flawed" and can spend a lot of time focusing on what's wrong with you and how you need or can change it. Also, it can lead to mental health issues such as anxiety, depression, eating disorders, obsessive-compulsive disorders, and substance use disorders. BDD can drive a person to self-harm or have thoughts of suicide. If you have thoughts of self-harm, seek immediate help by calling 911 or going to the emergency room.

How you see yourself and feel about your looks can take many forms. Here are a few examples:
- Taking something about your body that you think is a flaw and spending excessive amounts of time thinking about it.
- Compare your appearance to others.
- Repeatedly check your appearance or ask for other's feedback.
- Avoid taking photos or seeing your reflection.
- Always changing your appearance such as hair color, hair styles, tanning, clothes, etc.
- Frequently taking selfies or using filters on pictures of yourself.
- Changing your appearance frequently (tanning, changing your hairstyle, changing clothes, etc.).
- Worrying or having panic attacks from worrying about what you think others are saying about your appearance.

- Feeling shame or disgust towards your body.
- Calling yourself names such as "ugly," "hideous," "disgusting," "abnormal," "weird," "unattractive."
- Compulsively grooming yourself such as picking pimples, pulling hairs, or plucking.
- Avoid social situations where you feel like people will judge your appearance.
- Continuous cosmetic surgery to "fix" problems in your body.
- Thoughts of hurting yourself or suicide.

Transfer Addictions

"For me, getting enough sleep, drinking lots of water, having a healthy diet, and staying away from alcohol are musts. It's so boring, I know, but doing those things really helps."

— Jessica Biel

As with any addiction, it is very *common* when taking the primary addiction away, another addiction will take its place. You may already have more than an addiction to food. A common addiction you may have is spending or shopping, especially for new clothes. It's an exciting journey to buy new smaller clothes and it may be hard to stop buying, especially if you've been wearing the old clothes for a while.

Addictions are *not* a healthy way to live. When practiced in excess they can cause other problems in your life. Think about it. Go to a restaurant and observe the other tables. How many people are actually talking to each other and how many are absorbed in their phones? What about young children? How many would prefer to play on their iPad rather than toys or playing outside?

With the innovation of technology society has become more impatient. People want instant gratification. The internet allows you to have information access right at your fingertips and get answers instantly. And what about fast food? In just a few minutes you can have a hot meal in your hands. You're tired. You want food quick. Can drive-thru or take out become an addiction? Absolutely.

Get support if you can't get your addiction under control. Consider going to a 12-step meeting either in person or online. Find other support groups too. Talk to others who are struggling with the same things as you. Post in your Facebook bariatric support groups. Others may have found some helpful solutions. Know when you need professional help to deal with your addictions. Seek counseling.

Here are Some of the Most Common Addictions. Circle the Ones you Feel like you Might have an Addiction.

Alcohol, vapes, shopping, anorexia nervosa, purging, excessively weighing, cigars, smoking, food, illicit drugs, relationships, Adderall, Xanax, caffeine, opiates, Ambien, coffee, candy, Hydrocodone, online shopping, amazon, eBay, Etsy, Offer-up, Facebook, pain pills, heroin, fentanyl, weed, sweets, clothes, meth, sex, gym, attention, bar hopping, baking/decorating cookies, gambling, Starbucks, scrolling the internet, gaming, politics, cooking, Benzodiazepines, Tylenol PM's, chocolate, gardening, crocheting, Oxycodone, spending money, vomiting after eating, scratch off tickets, casino, thrift shopping, grocery shopping, Pinterest, codependency, THC edibles, Shien.

What addictions do you have?

_____

_____

_____

How have these addictions affected your life?

_____

_____

_____

What other things can you do except turn towards your addiction?

_____

_____

_____

Trauma

"The hard days are what make you stronger."
— Aly Raisman

Trauma and abuse can be physical, mental, or sexual, but the outcome is still the same. Whether trauma happened to you or you witnessed trauma, your emotions will be left in a mess, and you feel violated. These feelings don't go away until you deal with the trauma. Learning practical coping skills will help. If you can't move past the trauma, even if it happened 20 years ago, you should seek professional help.

As an adult, trauma could still affect you. People who have suffered from trauma and abuse are more likely to develop an eating disorder. Binging is quite common in people who have a history of abuse. Emotional eating caused from trauma attempts to cover or bury the pain inside of you, only it's an *illusion*. The pain is still there. It will come up again and again.

Thus, the cycle begins of eating and numbing. You will continue this cycle until you face and deal with the trauma. Only then are you able to compartmentalize the trauma and move on. The desire to numb the pain will then leave you. One problem is that you may not want to relive and *feel* the pain of the trauma again. Talk to a professional about other ways to move past the pain of the trauma.

Trauma can affect you by either something happening directly to you or you have been exposed to the trauma. It can be from violence, death, grief, natural disasters, illness, war, job loss, or finances. These traumas affect your emotional and mental self.

Be kind to past versions of yourself that didn't know the things you know now. That feeling of being out of control is hard in itself. You may wish there may have been something you could have done more or even to prevent the trauma. You may even blame yourself.

IT IS NOT YOUR FAULT!!!
TRAUMA NEVER IS!

Unhealed Trauma

Unhealed trauma can affect you in many ways that you may not have realized where it came from. You may be "stuck" in the trauma or even blame yourself. To move on, you must *heal* from the pain. If you are still in an abusive situation or relationship, you will not be able to heal. What prevents you from leaving?

Abusive people make you feel that it's all you or everything is your fault. Know that it's *not* your fault! That person may be controlling, manipulative, or even a narcissist. They may isolate you from your friends and family. Keep your eyes open and get help. *Get out!!*

Some of the Symptoms of Unhealed Trauma Include:

1. Chronic headache, pain, or fatigue
2. Hair pulling or skin picking
3. Addiction
4. Chronic or heightened states of fight/flight mode
5. Fatigue
6. Hypervigilance
7. Lack of trust
8. Anger
9. PTSD

PTSD

"Beware of destination addiction – a preoccupation with the idea that happiness is in the next place, the next job and with the next partner. Until you give up the idea that happiness is somewhere else, it will never be where you are."

— Robert Holden, Ph.D.

Post-traumatic stress disorder is the result of trauma. It affects you today as if it just happened. When you are triggered by things, smells, sounds or others that remind you of the past trauma, you will react as if that trauma is happening right now. You could have flashbacks in your mind of the event. An example for military persons that served in war would be hearing fireworks. This can trigger them right back to the battlefield.

Symptoms of PTSD:

1. Sleep disturbance/Nightmares
2. Flashbacks
3. Anger outbursts
4. Feeling numb

5. Avoiding anything that reminds you of the trauma

Resolving Trauma

Trauma refers to your *response* following an event that psychologically overwhelms you, often resulting in shock, denial, and changes in the body, mind, and behavior. You need to make peace with your trauma and your perpetrators. This doesn't mean that you agree. It only means you need to let them leave your mind and move on. You have to accept what happened to you. Acceptance is just saying, "it is what it is." It is for YOU not them. It is for YOUR peace not to excuse what they did to you.

What trauma have you experienced?

_____
_____
_____

How has that trauma affected you throughout your life?

_____

_____

_____

Who do you blame for the trauma?

_____

_____

_____

If you are in current trauma, what keeps you stuck there?

_____

_____

_____

How can you get out?

_____

_____

_____

Triggers

"True self-discovery begins where your comfort zone ends."
— Adam Braun

What are triggers? Triggers happen in your mind when anything reminds you of past events that cause you to feel as though they are happening today, right now in the moment. It could be from a past trauma or anything arousing your senses...sight, smell, taste, hear or feel. You will have the *same* feelings, thoughts, and memories as you did before. Sometimes this can be too much for you to deal with if it's things you've never dealt with before. Then you will want to turn to food for comfort.

For example: you see a couple fighting might trigger you back into a bad relationship; you smell a certain cologne and it reminds you of your deceased father and the tears just begin to flow even though your father has been gone for several years; you taste something bad like spoiled milk and you remember having food poisoning; you hear a man yelling and you're reminded of the times your parents fought; you feel a certain fabric like satin and you remember wearing satin pajamas on your honeymoon to your now ex-.

Triggers can also be a reminder of good times, such as around food. Therefore, certain foods can be considered "love" foods. Eating or thinking about them will bring happy memories. These comfort foods might just be the ones you begin to crave. Be careful!

Food can also be used as a coping mechanism to deal with life's difficult situations. Turning to food is what got you in the place you are now, before surgery. You need to rely on your new coping skills and support systems.

Growing up what events happened to you that you used food to cover up your feelings?

_____
_____
_____

How did your family use food to cover up pain?

_____

_____

_____

What are your "love" foods?

_____

_____

_____

What sights, smells, tastes, sounds, trigger you to cause you to turn to food for comfort?

_____

_____

_____

Check all that you identify as triggers:

- ☐ Anger and frustration
- ☐ Bad breakups
- ☐ Bad relationships
- ☐ Bad weather/hurricanes/tornado's
- ☐ Being afraid
- ☐ Being alone
- ☐ Being bored
- ☐ Being bullied
- ☐ Being in a bad mood
- ☐ Being lonely
- ☐ Being on a very restrictive diet
- ☐ Being sick and craving comfort food
- ☐ Being yelled at
- ☐ Buffets
- ☐ Certain difficult people
- ☐ Cultural pressure
- ☐ Death and grief
- ☐ Eating out of a bag

- ☐ Eating while watching TV, on the computer or reading a book
- ☐ Eating out
- ☐ Excessive worrying
- ☐ Fairs and festivals
- ☐ Fatigue
- ☐ Feeling deprived
- ☐ Feeling left out
- ☐ Feeling like you need a treat
- ☐ Feeling sorry for yourself
- ☐ Fixating on food
- ☐ "Free food" at work
- ☐ Getting too hungry
- ☐ Going out to eat in places that have your binge foods
- ☐ Going to a movie
- ☐ Going to an amusement park
- ☐ Go to parties/weddings where there is a lot of food
- ☐ Going out with drinking and eating friends
- ☐ Having anxiety

- ☐ Holding in your emotions and using food for comfort
- ☐ Hunger pains
- ☐ Infidelity
- ☐ Jealousy
- ☐ Let yourself get too hungry
- ☐ Love foods
- ☐ Mindless distracted eating
- ☐ Negative people
- ☐ Negative thoughts and emotions
- ☐ Nighttime
- ☐ Not standing up for yourself
- ☐ Only have fast food options
- ☐ Overthinking about your problems
- ☐ People who lie
- ☐ People who manipulate
- ☐ Places with no healthy food options
- ☐ Portion control is difficult
- ☐ Restricting all day and waiting too late to eat
- ☐ Rewarding yourself
- ☐ Seasonal foods

- ☐ Seeing or smelling food
- ☐ Self-Esteem issues
- ☐ Sibling rivalry
- ☐ Skipping meals
- ☐ Snacks
- ☐ Someone reminding you of past trauma
- ☐ Stress
- ☐ Sweets
- ☐ Thinking you are hungry when you're not
- ☐ Tiredness
- ☐ Too much alcohol
- ☐ Too much bad food in the house
- ☐ Trauma
- ☐ Trigger foods
- ☐ Vacation
- ☐ Visiting friends and not having healthy food choices
- ☐ Watching others eat

ADD YOUR OWN:

1.

2.

3.

4.

5.

**Pain changes your life forever
But so does healing from it.**

scars.

i hope my scars never fade
completely. that way people
who see them will always know
that they have someone
they can talk to. my pain does
not need to define me
but it will refine me.
and there is no better story to tell
than that of a life changed by the
very fire that tried to take you.

— ullie-kaye

Part II -
Living the Bariatric Life

Chapter 5

Pre-Surgery

"It's about taking the time before food goes in your mouth to be aware: Am I aware that I'm eating this? And am I eating it because I'm hungry or because I need to soothe myself?"
— Valerie Bertinelli

Your STATS

Name: _____ Date: _____

Phone: _____ City/State: _____

Highest Weight (HW): _____ Age: _____
Sex: M   F

Lowest Weight (LW): _____   Height: _____

Current Weight (CW): ____ Goal weight (GW): _____

Surgery Date: _____   Type of surgery: _____

Measurements (Pre-Op)

Neck: _____ Arm: _____ Bust: _____

Under bust: _____ Waist: _____ Stomach: _____

Hips: _____ Thigh: _____ Calf: _____

Other Important Stats:

_____

_____

_____

What some of the bariatric community has said:

1. I got a date. Now what?
2. Surgery day is tomorrow morning. I'm excited, nervous, scared all at one.
3. What do I take to the hospital?
4. I'm worried about never eating normal food again.
5. It's normal to be concerned. If we weren't then I'd be concerned.
6. This operation is a last resort. You have no choice after it but to control yourself. After all there's a reason why we all got into this mess in the first place.
7. Even though I had complications I don't regret having the surgery.
8. I'd have zero complications.
9. I wish these problems would go away.
10. It could be a lot worse.
11. It's not brain surgery, it's stomach surgery.
12. It's not a quick fix.
13. Surgery is a tool…not a magic wand.

14. The surgery itself is the easy part.
15. I'm having a hard time dealing with this acid reflux.
16. I knew my skin would sag, but this is ridiculous!
17. This pre-op diet is killing me!
18. I just want real food.
19. I didn't think I could do it, but here I am killing it.
20. There are times I want to back out.
21. Losing weight before surgery is such a bonus.
22. I really need to focus on one day at a time.
23. Listen to your body.
24. Get everyone in the house onboard with eating healthier.
25. It takes a lifetime commitment.
26. My health and success is determined by me.
27. It's not an easy fix or the easy way out.
28. Don't compare yourself to others.
29. The surgery fixes the body and not the mind.
30. Take advantage of the gift and window we are given.

31. Only do the surgery if it's your decision.
32. Do this for you!
33. Take it one day at a time or one meal at a time or one minute at a time.
34. The surgery is just a tool.
35. Look at a menu before you go to a restaurant.
36. Remember that the reason you're doing this is to make your life better.
37. If you take the easy road and do the bare minimum, you will get the results that show the easy road.
38. I started my goals of improving myself when I was finally divorced.
39. I want to do so much.
40. Up your volume of water pre-surgery.
41. Give up carbonated beverages before surgery.
42. My goal is to get off all medication.
43. I need to get in all my protein, water, and vitamins.
44. Set those goals and smash them.

45. Think about what you want, where you want to be, and how you're going to get there.
46. Don't minimize your goals because of fear.
47. Just remember, you are in charge of your life and journey.

Helpful Pre-Surgery Tips:

1. Your taste buds will change so don't stock up on bariatric food such as protein shakes pre-op.
2. Get off caffeinate and carbonated drinks before surgery because of the bad headaches and withdrawals.
3. Start the habit of not drinking while eating and waiting 30 minutes after eating to drink now before surgery.
4. Be honest in your bariatric psychological evaluation.
5. Lose the recommended weight loss before surgery.
6. Pre-op process may take a while.
7. Be patient. It's a process and lifestyle change.
8. You don't need a "Last supper."
9. If weight loss surgery was the easy way out, they wouldn't put you through months of physical and mental preparation before even considering you as a candidate.

10. You'll gain weight if you don't get help with your mindset before the surgery, it's not just about portion control, it's a lifestyle change. Be aware of everything you put into your mouth including drinks.
11. It's *really* hard work and not some easy magical fix where you wake up thin.
12. It's a tool, yes if you can follow the rules of the lifestyle change you will lose the weight and keep it off.
13. Everyone's journey is different, and everyone is going to lose weight at a different rate.
14. It's normal to second guess your decision to have bariatric surgery.
15. Don't let fear cause you to back out.

How are you feeling about having the surgery?

_____
_____
_____

What second thoughts are you having?

_____

_____

_____

What other ways have you tried to lose weight?

_____

_____

_____

What fears do you have about having bariatric surgery?

_____

_____

_____

What positive things can you say to yourself about moving forward with the surgery?

_____

_____

_____

Pre-op Challenges

"Believe you can, and you are half-way there."
— Theodore Roosevelt

Pre-op Diet

While you are pre-op, don't try and find ways to eat whatever you want. You don't need a "last supper." There will be many foods you will once again be able to eat. You're having this surgery to be a better, healthier you which requires you to change your old habits.

The pre-op liquid diet is helping to shrink your liver and prepare you for what to expect after surgery. If you're thinking "I don't how I'm going to make it on this liquid diet" know that you *can* do it. You'll have to do it again after surgery. Please don't cheat on your liquid diet!

PLEASE...FOLLOW YOUR PLAN!

How are you feeling about the pre-op diet?

_____

_____

_____

What are your struggle with the pre-op diet?

_____

_____

_____

What did you learn during pre-op stage?

_____

_____

_____

What is something positive you can tell yourself to get through pre-op diet?

_____

_____

_____

Advice

"Just believe in yourself. Even if you don't, pretend that you do, and at some point, you will."

— Venus Williams

Everyone has advice to give including family, friends, bariatric patients, and non-bariatric patients. Know that you should listen but then make your *own* decisions. First and foremost, listen to your bariatric doctor and follow *your* plan. Everyone's journey is different and just because one person has experienced something doesn't mean you will.

With that being said, some advice can be helpful. It may be things that you didn't know or even think about. When in doubt, ask your bariatric team. They are there for you and want your success as much as you do. They are your best advocates.

It is good pre-surgery to work on your emotional eating. For your success, you should learn how *not* to turn to food for comfort. If you need to see a therapist, do so. Get yourself in good mental and physical shape. Stop smoking, drinking carbonated drinks, up your water intake, and speak to other bariatric patients. Really get a feel for the life you are getting ready to embark upon. This is *forever*...for the rest of your life.

Good Advice about Having Bariatric Surgery

1. Life after bariatric surgery is *hard*...but will get easier and is worth it.
2. The first 3 days – 1 week after surgery is the hardest. You may experience pain in your body from the gas that was put into your body during surgery. Walk, walk, walk. You may be filled with regret.
3. Always be prepared. Keep healthy food in the house. Make sure you have something you can eat if you have low blood sugar episodes.
4. Get rid of your bigger clothes as you shrink out of them. Part with them with love and bless

someone else. No need to hang onto them as it may normalize being that size again.

5. When you get bored with your eating choices get creative and look for recipes on Pinterest or Facebook bariatric groups.
6. Try to avoid difficult places until you get stronger. Bakeries, grocery stores, or restaurants can be very difficult temptations at first.
7. When going to a social event that will have food, go prepared. Keep a snack in your purse or car. Never go thinking there will be something there you can eat.
8. Restaurants (not all fast-food ones) should always have something you can eat. They should have soup or salad. Some people eat a child's meal. Others ask for a take-out box with their meal and pack half to go. That way the temptations will be lessened.
9. When discouraged, remember why you had the surgery.

10. Attention will increase. People that never spoke to you before may all of a sudden be very friendly. Fat shaming is real. This may make you angry.
11. Relationships may become strained. Your significant other may become jealous of your new body and changes. People who were your friends may suddenly become jealous and angry at your progress.
12. Turn to your support systems for help.

Things to Do

"My nutritionist says, 'If you bite it, write it.' Writing down "everything that you put in your mouth really helps. I don't count a damn calorie. But when I'm really trying to eat healthy, I write everything down. It really holds me accountable and puts me on a healthier path."

— Tyra Banks

Before Surgery

There are things to do before bariatric surgery and others to do along the way. Weigh and measure yourself after your first bariatric appointment. Then do the same the day of surgery, although it is common for the hospital to weigh you that morning. It is interesting to see your removed stomach, so ask your surgeon to take a picture of it.

After Surgery

Try not to weigh yourself every day but only once a week. Measuring yourself and monitoring the changes in how your clothes fit is a better option.

Taking pictures will make it easier to see along the way. Keeping a food journal is an important way to track what you're eating and drinking. It will also help you identify when you're at a stall if this is normal or your eating is off. There are many apps for your smartphone to help track everything from calories to water.

Seek help when struggling. Talk to other bariatric patients, share in bariatric Facebook groups, or consult with your bariatric team. You should never feel *alone* during this journey. Others who have gone through the same things you have, can help you get past your difficulties.

Bring to the Hospital

You're in a professional's hands, so don't worry. Keep patience, and everything will be fine.

What some of the bariatric community has said:

1. Gas-X
2. Phone charger
3. Comfy clothes
4. Robe
5. Slippers
6. Underwear
7. Socks
8. Deodorant
9. Lip balm
10. Shampoo
11. Conditioner
12. Hairbrush
13. Toothbrush
14. Toothpaste
15. Mouthwash

16. Pj's

17. In case you have a roommate, earbuds

18. Comfort items – Book, crossword puzzle book, laptop

19. Your best attitude to overcome any pain or discomfort

20. Patience!

If you have never been in the hospital, you will have many questions as to what to bring and expect. You may feel undue stress about going to the hospital and the surgery itself. Most people have a one-night stay. However, if you have complications your stay in the hospital may be longer.

Bring with you comfort items. Your own belongings will give you a sense of peace. If you need additional items, have someone bring it to you. Don't worry, hospitals are equipped to provide you with the necessities if you forget anything. It will be over sooner that you anticipate, so just *relax*.

How are you feeling about your upcoming surgery and hospital stay?

_____
_____
_____

What comfort items will you bring?

_____
_____
_____

What can you do to relieve your anxiety about surgery?

_____
_____
_____

Goals

"Whatever your goal for this year is, you can get there—as long as you're willing to be honest with yourself about the preparation and work involved."

— Oprah

Bariatric life is hard yet rewarding. It is important to recognize the goals and achievements you will have during your journey. Set a realistic goal weight before the surgery. Discuss with your bariatric team to make sure it is attainable. When you reach that goal, if you're happy where you are, that is great. If not, re-evaluate and set another goal weight. You can set 10 lbs. at a time if you want. The main thing is to set a goal that is attainable.

Get a goal outfit or search into the back of your closet and pull out an outfit you loved and would love to wear again. Periodically look at that outfit. Put it up to yourself and look in the mirror. Imagine yourself in that outfit. Then tell yourself, *"Soon…real soon."*

Set some fitness goals. Start small. You may want to walk to the mailbox and back. Each week add a little more to that goal. Who knows? You may one day run in a race? Dream! Allow yourself to dream *big*.

Set some short-term goals. Make small realistic goals that you can reach. It will be such an accomplishment when you achieve these goals. And then set some long-term goals. What are things you've always wanted to do, go, or become? The sky is the limit. Put it all down.

When you list a goal, especially a long-term goal, break it down into smaller parts. If cleaning your house is your goal, that can be overwhelming. Break it down room by room, then corners of the room and finally a surface area. That way you will see that every little step is attainable. Make sure to check off your list when you attain a goal. This will give you a feeling of accomplishment.

YOU WILL SUCCEED!!

SHORT-TERM GOALS:

1.

2.

3.

4.

LONG-TERM GOALS:

1.

2.

3.

4.

Complications

Don't get discouraged by what you're going through. Your time is coming. Be patient. Where you are is not where you are going to stay.

As with all surgeries, complications can happen. Do not let this discourage you from getting the surgery. It is good to be informed though. Listen to other bariatric patients but don't let their negatives influence your decision. Remember, *not* everyone will experience the exact same things. Below you will see an extended list of all possible complications of bariatric surgery.

All Procedures:
- Excessive bleeding
- Infection
- Adverse reactions to anesthesia
- Pneumonia
- Infection and bleeding at the surgical site
- Internal or excessive bleeding
- Lung or breathing problems
- Perforation and leak from the bowel

- Malabsorption of other nutrients
- Loose, sagging skin
- Blood clots
- Gastrointestinal bleeding or leaks
- Gallstones
- Failure to lose weight
- Intractable vomiting
- Death (0.1% - 2%)

Gastric Banding

- Band erosion
- Band slippage
- Band or port infections
- Esophageal dilation
- Port displacement
- Port disconnection

Gastric Bypass

- Stomal stenosis
- Marginal ulcers
- Anastomotic leak with peritonitis
- Small bowel obstruction
    - Internal hernia
    - Adhesions
- Staple line disruption
- Dumping syndrome
- Nutrient deficiencies
    - Calcium

- Iron
- Vitamin B12
- Folic acid

Vertical Sleeve Gastrectomy
- Excessive bleeding
- Infection
- Adverse reactions to anesthesia
- Blood clots
- Lung or breathing problems
- Leaks from the cut edge of the stomach

Longer Term Risks and Complications of Sleeve Gastrectomy Surgery can Include:
- Gastrointestinal obstruction
- Hernias
- Gastroesophageal reflux
- Low blood sugar (hypoglycemia)
- Malnutrition
- Vomiting
- Ulcers

Long-Term Health Complications of Weight-Loss Surgery can Include:
- Anemia due to a deficiency of iron or B12
- Neurological complications, such as memory loss or irritability from a lack of B12
- Bone and kidney disease due to changes in the way your body absorbs calcium and vitamin D

- Bowel obstruction
- Dumping syndrome, which leads to diarrhea, flushing, lightheadedness, nausea or vomiting
- Gallstones
- Hernias
- Low blood sugar, called hypoglycemia
- Malnutrition
- Ulcers
- Vomiting
- Acid reflux
- The need for a second, or revision, surgery, or procedure
- Rarely, death

Chapter 6

Post-Surgery

"If you take care of your body, it'll take care of you."
— Usher

What some of the bariatric community has said:

1. I can do this.
2. Even though I'm in pain, I will get through this.
3. I focus on one day at a time.
4. Be mindful to sip, sip, sip.
5. My new life has begun!
6. The lap band wasn't a permanent solution.
7. The day after surgery you will have great regrets.
8. Extreme pain is possible from one or more stitch or a drain tube.
9. I didn't realize I'd be in so much pain after surgery.

10. The first 6 weeks you will be filled with regret.
11. Taste buds change.
12. Drains after surgery are painful.
13. Life after lap band removal is totally different.
14. Walk often and lots to decrease painful gas.
15. Walking is the only way to feel any kind of relief.
16. Walk, walk, walk.
17. It takes willpower, diet, and exercise to work post-surgery.
18. My new stomach is just a tool. The real work still needs to be done by me.
19. Slow and steady wins the race.
20. Heating pad for the gas.
21. The first month's mental toll is hard.
22. I'm exhausted, overwhelmed, feel like crap, emotional, these gas pains suck and I'm feeling a little regret.
23. Honeymoon period doesn't last long.
24. Can only eat 5 bites of food.

25. Key to success: Stick to protein and water goals as long as you're losing.
26. You eat to live.
27. How small of portions I really eat.
28. Life is so much better.
29. No regrets, no regrets, no regrets
30. Chew! Chew! Chew!
31. The struggle of not eating and drinking together is real.
32. Slowing down to eat is hard for a fast eater.
33. Stick to YOUR plan.
34. Follow the rules for life.
35. Always eat protein first.
36. Slow down your eating.
37. Two things I'm working on is chewing to an applesauce consistency and slowing down eating.
38. Some can use straws, and some can't.
39. Chew to a puree.
40. It's hard to follow all the rules.

41. I never realized how important taking vitamins were.
42. Remember the before.
43. Remember the why you decided to get the surgery.
44. Be honest with yourself.
45. It's a process that takes time.
46. Moderation is key.
47. Don't get complacent.
48. During the "honeymoon" phase stay strict and try the hardest.
49. Don't pick up old habits.
50. Just because you aren't hungry, eat anyway.
51. Take those vitamins.
52. The costs of the vitamins and other medications you need are expensive.
53. Take your complex vitamin, calcium, and biotin.
54. I didn't realize by not taking my vitamins I'd get and look sick.

55. My dilemma is that I can no longer take big pills because they make me gag.
56. I take my vitamins like clockwork and I'm feeling good.
57. May never be able to gulp water down.
58. That if I don't drink all my water, I can get dehydrated.
59. How much I miss chugging water.
60. Drink sips of water all day to prevent dehydration.
61. Carbs in moderation don't work for me.
62. Beware of slider foods.
63. Don't start on the slider foods.
64. Microwave can dry out meat.
65. That I'd have to eat a snack every 3 hours.
66. Certain food smells can make me sick.
67. Just because you liked certain foods before you may not now.
68. I am sensitive to anything sweet.
69. Food will taste much spicier.

70. I wish I made more of my own broth for that stage.
71. Use measuring cups instead of a scale for food. It's about volume.
72. That I wouldn't be hungry after.
73. The full feeling only lasts an hour or so.
74. Some foods I used to love before surgery I can't stand the taste of after surgery.
75. Sensitivity to spicy and acidic foods.
76. Taste buds are weird.
77. Crunchie ice was a life saver after surgery.
78. Cannot drink alcohol the same again.
79. May be able to eat anything in moderation.
80. I thought sugar would make me sick.
81. Meats are hard to digest.
82. Just because I CAN eat something doesn't mean that I SHOULD.
83. Food would no longer be my friend.
84. Slider foods can be dangerous.
85. Enjoy the journey and experiment with different foods.

86. Eat for the body you want and not for the body you have.
87. Papaya enzymes is supposed to help break down food that may get stuck.
88. Our new pouch is sacred space. Treat it that way by feeding it protein enriched food.

Post-op Diet

Your desire to change must be greater than your desire to stay the same.

1) Follow your doctor's plan as it will vary from program to program.
2) Generally, you will start with all liquids and slowly advance to solid food over several weeks.
3) Post-op diet is very similar to the pre-op diet.
4) Exercise or walk when you can.
5) Stick to the stages of recovery:
    - Thin or clear liquids
    - Full liquids
    - Pureed food
    - Soft food
    - Regular food
    - Maintenance
6) Don't rush the healing process. It takes time for your body to heal from major surgery.
7) Follow the chewing and drinking rules.
8) Don't cheat! You are only hurting yourself!

You will have to make it work as your stomach is altered and you will have no choice. Your pouch won't be able to handle a lot of food and you can really harm your pouch if you cheat after surgery. Let your new stomach heal properly.

So, if you fail to plan, you're planning to fail. Life after bariatric surgery is a *lifestyle* change. You won't be able to eat like you could before. That's the purpose of the surgery! If you follow the rules, the weight will come off.

This is the most amazing tool anyone can be given for weight loss! If you emotionally eat, you will still emotionally eat if you haven't changed your mindset. Seek professional help if it's more than you can handle. It's up to *you* to keep yourself motivated and stay on track for a healthier you!

What pre-op diet stages did you have the most difficulty with?

_____

_____

_____

How can you make sure to keep your diet in check?

_____

_____

_____

What are you feeling about your post-op diet?

_____

_____

_____

Rules

"If you want to accomplish anything in life, you can't just sit back and hope it will happen. You've got to make it happen."

— Chuck Norris

FOLLOW THE RULES!!!
THEY ARE FOR LIFE!!!

Rules are in place to make sure you have a healthy bariatric life. You cannot go through this life-changing surgery and expect to eat the way you did before. Your body will remind you to slow down, take small bites, and not drink and eat at the same time. It's a learning process you will learn quick. Be gentle on yourself.

Bariatric life is *not* the easy way out. There are many rules you need to follow that may seem uncomfortable or the opposite of what you've always done. These rules are for life and not just during weight loss.

But they are put into place for a reason. Some of the rules you can or cannot decide to follow. Your success rate will be greater if you follow *all* the rules. Also, each bariatric office will have their own rules. It is best to ask them any questions you may have regarding the rules.

Rules to Follow:

1. Eat your protein first. You won't be able to eat much, and protein will keep you full longer. Also, protein will help with losing hair.
2. Drink or sip water throughout the day. Stay hydrated.
3. Take small bites of food. And…chew, chew, chew.
4. Chew your food 21 times before you swallow.
5. Try different protein drinks. You never know what you will enjoy drinking.

6. Never return to drinking carbonated beverages such as soft drinks. This could eventually stretch out your new stomach.
7. If you drink alcohol, a very small amount will be enough. Your new stomach will not be able to handle much alcohol at all and will process it differently.
8. Don't drink 30 minutes before or 30 minutes after a meal. Don't drink while you eat. This is important so your food stays in your stomach longer and is not being washed through by liquids. You will consume a lot more calories that way.
9. Learn to notice when you're full. Don't push past that point or you may throw up. Some people burp, nose's run, sneeze, sigh, cough, or get hiccups when they are full.
10. Your clothes sizes will change quickly. Don't go out and buy a lot of clothes until you reached your goal weight. You may shop at 2nd hand stores to get you by.

11. Don't weigh every day. Once a week is a better choice.
12. Have your support system in place.
13. Exercise as soon as you can. It will help with sagging skin as you lose.
14. You might be cold all the time because you lost your insulation.
15. Your tailbone can hurt after losing your butt padding.
16. Your hair will fall out. It's part of the process of rapid weight loss.
17. Know when to get professional help. Your new bariatric lifestyle may require facing why you turn to food for comfort. A professional therapist can help you with this process.

Rules I need to follow that may be hard:

_____

_____

_____

Rules I don't understand why I must follow:

_____

_____

_____

What is my resistance to following these rules?

_____

_____

_____

Vitamins

"When you are a warrior for your body, you search out every good thing there is to fill it with – every nutrient, every vitamin, every thought, every belief. You love your body, and you thank your body in the morning and bless it throughout the day."

— Debbie Ford

Bariatric surgery changes your body and digestion. You will absorb fewer nutrients that your body gets from food. To prevent nutritional deficiencies, you will need to take vitamin and mineral supplements daily for the rest of your life. It is recommended that you initiate vitamin and mineral supplements after bariatric surgery. But check with your surgeon's office to confirm.

Vitamins and minerals are needed because you are eating smaller amounts of food since the size of the stomach has been reduced. It's critical to review your vitamin and mineral levels regularly. Check with your dietitian or bariatric team to determine if your vitamin and mineral routine is meeting your needs. Vitamins are available in pills, liquids, chewable, gummies, dissolving pills and patches.

Vitamins or Minerals that are Recommended:

Multivitamin - Needs to be chewable or liquid for the first several months after surgery. Choose a chewable complete multivitamin with iron.

Calcium – May need to take calcium several times a day and without other vitamins and minerals. Calcium citrate is the preferred form of calcium. Take calcium with meals.

Additional Vitamins and Minerals you may Take:

B12 - Plays an essential role in red blood cell formation, cell metabolism, nerve function and DNA production. Good for an increase in energy.

Biotin - An important part of enzymes in the body that break down substances like fats, carbohydrates, and others. Biotin deficiency can cause thinning of the hair and a rash on the face.

Collagen - Protein responsible for healthy joints and skin elasticity, or stretchiness.

D - Nutrient that helps build and maintain healthy bones and regulate cellular functions in the body, regulation of muscle contractions, and conversion of blood glucose (sugar) into energy.

Iron - An important mineral that helps maintain healthy blood. A lack of iron is called iron-deficiency anemia.

Magnesium - Is required for the proper growth and maintenance of bones, the proper function of nerves, muscles, and many other parts of the body. In the stomach, magnesium helps neutralize stomach acid and moves stools through the intestine.

What supplements do you take every day?

_____
_____
_____

Water

Keep calm and drink water.

Water helps to flush toxins, waste, and weight from your body. It keeps your organs healthy and working properly. Water helps your heart pump blood more efficiently through your body and is a necessity for a healthy life.

Work on your water volume pre-surgery. After bariatric surgery, water is a requirement. Drinking enough water in a day can help prevent dehydration. There are many ways to enjoy water. Add flavored packets to your water to make it more appealing.

Count your water intake! In the beginning it is hard to get in all your water requirements but track it anyway. Even if you can't gulp water like before surgery, you can still enjoy it and get enough in. Sip all fluids. Sip, sip, sip!

Always carry a water bottle with you. That makes it easier to get in your required water intake amount. Don't drink water or any fluids 30 minutes before and after a meal. This will prevent food from being flushed through. Also, doing so may make your food come up and you can vomit.

How do you guarantee you're staying hydrated?
_____
_____
_____

What flavors have you tried or want to try added to your water?
_____
_____
_____

Food and Drinks

"Your diet is a bank account. Good food choices are good investments."

— Bethenny Frankel

Increasing your protein intake will keep you full longer. Add unflavored protein powder to food or drinks. Adding cheese to foods can also increase your protein intake. Get creative and find ways to increase your protein like choosing protein rich snacks.

Food can get stuck if not chewed up enough to go down. It feels like it's lodged belong your sternum. You will also feel very nauseous. One of the best ways to get past it is to drink water. It will make you automatically throw up and you will get instant relief.

Taste buds can change daily. One day you may enjoy one food and other days you don't. Keep trying along the way. Your taste buds *may* allow certain foods again. For some, spicy foods can be an issue causing pain and acid reflux.

You will never be able to drink alcohol the same way as before surgery. Your body absorbs differently now. Only a very small amount of alcohol will hit your system harder than before. Be careful and sip your alcohol so you can stay conscience of how your body is reacting.

What foods help you feel full longer?

_____

_____

_____

What foods can you no longer tolerate? What happens?

_____

_____

_____

How does your body respond to alcohol?

_____

_____

_____

Chapter 7

Living in Wellness

"Change happens when the pain of staying the same is greater than the pain of change."

— Tony Robbins

What some of the bariatric community has said:

1. I have to remind myself I've come a very long way and we are humans that need to allow ourselves some grace.
2. Give it a couple of months, it gets easier day by day, then one day you wake up and feel normal and the rest is history. You won't even remember the dark days.
3. Losing weight will be fun when you have to buy a whole new wardrobe.
4. This journey has been amazing!!
5. Building muscle = weight gain.

6. I love the person I've become because I fought hard to become her.
7. Whatever makes you feel the sun from the inside out…Chase that.
8. I do lots of walking, yoga and core strengthening exercises.
9. I got a personal trainer to help me at the gym.
10. Wall/reg Pilates, and lazy girl stretching videos on YouTube are what I do.
11. I hate exercise. What can I do?
12. Is exercise really necessary to lose weight?
13. Exercise is too hard.
14. You still have to put the work in.
15. Not to read all the negative posts.
16. It's all a learning curve.
17. Journey is all consuming.
18. You are stronger than you know.
19. Exercise makes my body hurt.
20. It's a forever struggle with no finish line, not even goal weight.

21. To get the results you want, eat right and workout.
22. My success and health are still determined by my choices.
23. Road is not easy but is worth it. Hitting goal weight is not the finish line.
24. In the middle of the hard years, I made sure to double down on my good habits so I would at least maintain and not gain.
25. I'm scared to move into maintenance. I've always been able to lose, but not maintain and keep it off.
26. Maintenance for me is where the real work begins.
27. My new goal is to maintain.
28. Embrace the journey.
29. Realize that the actual feeling of hunger is not harmful.
30. When hungry, realize that your next meal is that far away.

The Process

"Staying in shape and staying fit is so important in my life just because of all the things I want to do."
— Melissa Joan Hart

Congratulations! You have learned about the mental part, emotional eating, your relationship with food, and healthy coping skills. Being aware is the *first* step to making positive and lasting changes. With this knowledge, you can now make a conclusive decision about whether you will proceed with having bariatric surgery. You may still be feeling many emotions, but you have all the emotional insight and tools you need to be successful.

As you know, having bariatric surgery is *not* a magic fix. And it's *not* the easy way out. Bariatric surgery should be an option when all else fails. If you are extremely obese or just have a little to lose but have tried every way possible, then it's a great option available to you. One perk is that it is permanent which means that you will have permanent weight loss and health results…*If* you continue to follow the rules.

In the final chapters of the book, you will learn some truth about life after bariatric surgery. But take it with a grain of salt as not everyone experiences all that will be discussed. Don't let it scare you away. It's better to be informed and know about what could happen. Knowledge is power!

YOU CAN DO THIS!!!

Life after Bariatric Surgery

"Staying in shape and staying fit is so important in my life just because of all the things I want to do."
— Melissa Joan Hart

Restriction will vary some days. Make sure you are getting in enough protein. If you're still hungry, drink water. Sometimes hunger can mask as thirst. Then wait awhile to see if you still feel hungry. Being satisfied and being full are two totally different things. Learn to identify the differences.

Develop Healthy Lifestyle Habits.

When you have developed healthy lifestyle habits it will be easier to get through difficult times without turning to food. Being relaxed, well rested and physically strong will help you to be better prepared to handle all things that may come up in your life. If you aren't at peak performance, you will have a difficult time handling the challenges that come with the bariatric life.

Healthy Lifestyle Habits.

- **Exercise Daily.** Any amount of physical activity can boost your mood and energy levels. It can also reduce stress. The key is to find an exercise you enjoy.
- **Try to get 8 Hours of Sleep Every Night.** When you are tired and not feeling rested, often your body will crave something sweet to give you a quick energy boost. Getting plenty of rest will help with appetite control and reduce food cravings.
- **Make Relaxation a Priority.** Take at least 30 minutes a day to relax and unwind. This is great for your mental health. It could be relaxing in a quiet room or a hot bubble bath. This is your time to take a break from your responsibilities, decompress, and recharge your batteries. Many

people do this after work when they first get home.

- **Reach out to Others.** Close relationships and social activities are a good way to stay connected with others. You are not alone! Choose your circle of friends carefully. Seek positive people who will enhance your life. This will help protect you from the negative effects of stress in your life or theirs.

What do you do to relax or decompress?

_____

_____

_____

Instead of turning to food when stressed, what can you do instead?

_____

_____

_____

What are some healthy lifestyle habits you have?

_____

_____

_____

What healthy lifestyle habits can you add?

_____

_____

_____

Exercise

"For me, exercise is more than just physical – it's therapeutic."

— Michelle Obama

What is your goal after bariatric surgery? If it's to improve your health and enhance longevity, losing weight by changing your diet and having bariatric surgery is not enough. It is also important to understand the significance of increasing your level of physical activity.

Many health benefits are only achievable by elevating your heart rate, feeling some shortness of breath, and working to a light sweat. There are currently no wonder drugs or machines to perform these exercises for you. Therefore, it's up to you to embrace and change the level of physical activity in your life.

After bariatric surgery, you may not feel like exercising at first. Take your time and add exercise in slowly. Implementing healthy exercise habits is a key element for long-term success.

In addition to helping you lose weight, exercise stimulates the production of endorphins, the "feel good" hormones. Exercise also helps keep your bone tissue dense and strong, increases strength and balance, boosts energy, and improves your quality of life.

Research has shown that bariatric patients who exercise three or more times per week, for a minimum of 30 minutes, lost an additional 12% of their excess weight in six months. If you focus on exercise soon after surgery, you will likely find it very rewarding. As the weight falls off, your capacity for exercise changes dramatically, with significant improvements on a week-by-week basis.

Benefits of Exercise

- Reduces the risk of certain cancers, stroke, diabetes, and heart disease

- Improves self-confidence, energy, mood, and sleep
- Improves mental alertness and prevents dementia

3 Types of Exercises

Knowing you need exercise in order to gain great health benefits is a start. Understanding which exercises to do and how long you should perform them is the next step. There are three main types of exercise that impacts your body in different ways. A well-balanced exercise program should include some exercise from each category. Start slowly and work up to the recommended goals gradually.

Flexibility Exercises

Anaerobic exercise will tone your muscles through stretching and can prevent muscle and joint problems later in life. This should include a warm-up and cool-down period for your other exercises. Set a goal to do 10 to 20 minutes of flexibility exercises or stretching daily.

Cardiovascular Exercise

Aerobic exercise uses your large muscles and can be continued for long periods. It is any exercise that raises your heart rate to a level where you can still talk, but you start to sweat a little. Cardiovascular exercises drive your body to use oxygen more efficiently and deliver maximum benefits to your heart, lungs, and circulatory system. At least 20 minutes of cardiovascular exercise include: walking, jogging, swimming, and biking. Three or four days a week is a good place to start to maintain fitness. Any movement is good, even house or yard work. But if your goal is to lose weight, you will need to do some form of aerobic exercise for at least 30 minutes five or more days a week.

Strength-building Exercises

A form of anaerobic exercise that does not have cardiovascular (heart, lung, and blood circulation) benefits, but will makes your muscles and bones stronger is strength-building. These exercises require short, intense exertion. Strength-building exercise also increases your metabolism (how fast you burn calories) because muscles use calories for energy even when your body is at rest. By increasing the size of your muscles, you are burning more calories all of the time, not only when you are actively exercising. In addition, if you strength-train regularly, you will find that your body looks leaner and you will lose fat. Strength-building exercises should be done two to three times a week for best results. Always warm up your muscles for five to 10 minutes before you begin. This applies for lifting any type of weight or before performing any resistance exercises.

Exercise Prevents Loss of Bone and Muscle Mass

When the body is in a state of stress and trying to fight starvation and malnutrition, it hoards fat. What this means for you is that after your surgery, your body will burn muscle mass *before* fat. You must emphasize to your body that your muscles are needed through regular, daily exercise. Education is needed.

This idea is similar with calcium stored in your bones. Strong bones require calcium, phosphorous and other nutrients in addition to weight-bearing exercise. You may tend to have strong bones already because carrying extra weight makes every movement a weight-bearing exercise.

When major, rapid weight loss occurs and adequate mineral supplementation is lacking, the body may take needed nutrients out of the bones, and this makes osteoporosis (weak, fragile bones) more likely. To prevent this, perform at least 30 minutes a day of aerobic exercise and weight-bearing exercise. Devote attention to the whole body, including working on upper-body strength.

Tips for Sticking to Your Exercise Program

Here are some tips to help you make a long-term commitment to exercise. The key to sticking with exercise is finding something you enjoy. It could be walking, jogging, running, dancing, swimming, biking, climbing or many other activities you can do.

Improving your movement is important to shape up while you lose weight. You will tone and possibly have less hanging skin. A good workout will also strengthen your willpower and resolve. You are less likely to mindlessly eat something you shouldn't eat.

Look at Exercise like a Necessity

Treat your exercise routine like a prescription you must take daily, and you'll have more success. You do not have to like exercise, but you need to do it to stay healthy. It will also help you to lose weight.

Look for Local Opportunities

Find out what types of classes your local gym is offering. Does your hospital offer water exercise classes for people with arthritis? Is there a gentle yoga class offered at the recreational center? Explore new types of exercise and find one that you enjoy.

Change up your Routine

If you used to love to walk, but now are bored with it, try a simple change in your walking routine. Sometimes, just changing the direction of your route can make all the difference. Find new places to go walking, change the time of day, or walk your dog.

Find a Buddy

Let's face it, it helps to have someone to nudge you and make you go the extra mile, especially when it comes to exercise. Find a friend, a neighbor or personal trainer to meet you at the gym or in the park.

Find your Rhythm

Listen to music or books on tape, or practice meditation while you exercise. With something to occupy your brain, a normally tedious routine exercise, like 15 minutes on a stationary bike, will not seem so long.

Participate in Group Sports

You don't need to join a soccer team but participating in a group activity increases the chance you'll stick to it. Choose a water exercise, yoga or stretching class. Pick places and times where there are other people who are actively involved in exercise.

Know what Makes you Give up the Program

If boredom makes you give up, stay interested by changing types of exercise and times. If going on vacation throws you off your fitness plan, try incorporating exercise into your vacation.

Make a Schedule

If you don't put exercise into your daily schedule, most likely you will do everything but exercise. Schedule specific activities on specific days, like walking 20 minutes on Monday and a yoga class on Tuesday.

Use a Workout Log

Write down the exercise you do and see how you have improved. Just like weight loss, sometimes you don't see the scale drop, but the inches seem to melt away. It is difficult to keep up with exercise when you do not see the results. Write down the number of repetitions, the weight used, the length of walk, the time, and other data so you can see improvement.

Stay Active Between Workouts

Walk as much as possible between workouts. Park farther away. Get off the bus a couple of stops early. Always keep a good pair of walking shoes in your car, so if you have unexpected time, you can take a walk.

Find an Exercise that Works for You

Don't have enough energy to perform 30 minutes of exercise? Does joint pain limit your activity level? Don't give up. Even three to five minutes of light activity is something you should be able to complete without aggravating your pain. It may not be ideal, but any activity or movement can help. With time, you may even be able to build your endurance and strength little by little.

Make Exercise a Habit in your Life

The level of physical activity in your life should be a part of your daily routine. Often, changing your behavior, even when for the better, can be a challenging task. Even harder is trying to break the habits you learn at an early age. Most people experience the endless repetition of stepping forward and backward while attempting to change their routine.

Other external factors, such as busy schedules, family dynamics or even bad weather, can also be barriers. Remember, never be disappointed when you find yourself falling backward into old habits. Simply recognize it, remind yourself of your goals and try again for a healthier life. Get up, dust off your knees, and go on. You can do it!!

How do you feel about exercise? Explain.

_____

_____

_____

What types of activities do you enjoy that encourage exercise?

_____

_____

_____

What exercises can you incorporate into your journey?

_____

_____

_____

Maintenance

"What I know for sure is this: The big secret in life is that there is no big secret. There are no back doors, no free rides. There's just you, this moment, and a choice."

— Oprah

To realize when you are in maintenance can be hard for you. Before surgery have you ever been in maintenance? If so, how long did it last? Most people are used to always gaining or losing weight.

Maintenance can be a slippery slope. You may try adding back into your diet, foods you loved before. It is trial and error. To be successful in maintenance, you must maintain what you are eating and doing, while monitoring your weight.

Weigh only once a week and give yourself a limit of 5 pounds gained. Most days you will be up or down a few pounds. If you go over the 5-pound limit, look at what you've been eating. Tighten up where you can. You will love living in maintenance because the focus shifts from always wanting to lose more weight to being happy with where you are.

Plus, you can now buy clothes that you know you will always be able to fit in. No more multiple sizes in the closet. You will have clothes for all seasons that fit! Just grab and go!

How do you feel about being in maintenance?
_____
_____
_____

How will you maintain your weight loss?
_____
_____
_____

What food have you reintroduced since being in maintenance?
_____
_____
_____

Chapter 8

Lifestyle Benefits

Success is more than a number on the scale.

What some of the bariatric community has said:

1. Reflections in a building window are always a surprise.
2. Having my doctor say, "You are at goal weight."
3. Feeling comfortable in my body.
4. Get my confidence back.
5. Love how I look in clothes.
6. Being reminded that I look normal.
7. Getting a tattoo.
8. Reaching a healthy BMI.
9. It's not just the weight you lose, but the life you gain.
10. I'm no longer pre-diabetic.

11. I no longer snore.

12. I don't get acne anymore.

13. I can wrap a towel around myself.

14. I can shop in any store.

15. I don't look at weight limits on furniture.

16. I can go down a slide or on a swing.

17. I can run with my son.

18. I can ride a bike.

19. I can stand for long periods and my body doesn't hurt.

20. I can take a flight of stairs and not be winded.

21. My feet and ankles don't hurt.

22. I can wear heels.

23. I am more confident personally and professionally.

24. People go out of their way to be nice to me.

25. I can cross my legs in the car or on a chair.

26. Getting up off the ground easily.

27. Being able to lean over the washing machine to get the clothes at the bottom.

28. Bending over to tie my shoes.

29. I can comfortably fit in a plane seat & buckle my seat belt.
30. My things don't touch the door in my car.
31. I'm not embarrassed to ride in other people's cars.
32. My underwear won't stay up.
33. Not worrying about breaking the folding chair.
34. I have so much more energy.
35. I've had to learn how to reward myself without turning to food.
36. Non-food rewards are the best!
37. I look forward to rewarding myself for all of my hard work.
38. Who would have thought that I didn't need to turn to food for good reasons?
39. That I would be freed from being in a trapped fat body.
40. There will be many NSV (Non-scale victories).
41. That I'd never be hungry again.
42. Should have done it years ago.

43. How wonderful and lifechanging this journey would be.
44. Need to look for the positives.
45. Life is not over. It's just beginning!
46. That it's all worth it…All of it!
47. I may be a slow loser…but I'm not done yet.
48. Don't be so worried. It all works out in the end.
49. It's not easy but it's worth it.
50. Wish I would have done it sooner.
51. You will enjoy wearing tighter fitting clothes.
52. Baggy clothes will no longer feel comfortable.
53. You will finally love how your body feels and looks.
54. You can wear shirts tucked in.
55. After losing weight my bladder pressure is gone. I can now sleep through the night without waking up to go to the bathroom.
56. I'm in love with my new body.
57. I can't express my gratitude enough to my bariatric surgeon and staff.

58. I'm one-year post-op! I'm filled with pure gratitude.
59. I will forever be grateful for my new life!
60. I'd have an inner fatty bitch.
61. Seems easier to get pregnant after surgery.
62. How sexy I was going to be.
63. Should have done this sooner.
64. You will enjoy food again but in smaller quantities.
65. Waking up every day is such a joy.
66. It's all worth it. Every tear, frustration, moment of regret – worth it!

NSV's
(Non-scale victories)

"Victory belongs to the persevering."
— Napoleon Bonaparte

Are you seeing results? Is the scale moving? Do you have a negative relationship with the scale? Only focusing on weight loss *can* be discouraging. Don't let the scale define you. Looking at other areas you can define success will make you feel more confident and feeling better about yourself.

NSV's (Non-scale victories) are the extras that come along with bariatric surgery and weight loss. In addition to weight loss, there will be many little "bonuses" that you will have. Some are expected, while others will surprise you. These NSV's are perks to your new life after bariatric surgery.

There will be things you can do now that you may not thought you would *ever* be able to do again.

Or you will be totally amazed at what you can do. Enjoy them all! Feel free to add your own.

Non-scale Victories to Celebrate: (Stanborough, 2021)

1. Your clothes fit better than they used to

Judge your success by how your clothes are fitting. If they are move comfortable, your efforts are very likely paying off.

2. You can do more of the things you love

Physical activity doesn't have to take place in a gym. If you're on the path to a healthier life, you may find that your new habits are making it easier for you to get out and do things you enjoy more often. Playing with your children or pets, working in your garden, dancing to a favorite tune, or taking a brisk walk are all activities to celebrate.

3. You have more energy

An increase in energy is one NSV's that you get from eating healthier and losing weight.

4. Your sleep has improved

If your new activity and healthy eating habits have changed your weight, you may be sleeping more soundly at night.

5. You've reached a fitness milestone

If you're moving more than you used to, you'll probably notice changes in your fitness levels the longer you stick with it.

6. Your mind is sharper

When you change your diet, exercise more often, and lose weight in the process, your thinking skills are likely to improve.

7. Your skin looks better

Healthy eating and regular exercise improve the health of your whole body. But research shows that eating lots of fruits and vegetables may produce benefits that show up on your skin.

8. You've lost inches

Exercising along with weight loss can change your measurements. The scale will *not* reflect your inches lost.

9. Your coping mechanisms are healthier

You've learned healthy ways to stop emotional eating. This is a victory worth celebrating.

10. You're in less physical pain

Losing weight reduces the stress on the joints in your body thus causing less joint pain.

11. Your mood is improved

Another non-scale victory may be an improvement in your mood.

12. Your medical markers are getting better

If you've made healthy changes to your diet and exercise routines, a doctor's visit may show that important health markers like **blood pressure** and **blood sugar** are improving. People who lose weight because of a health concern often lose more weight at first and keep it off over time.

13. You have new sources of social support

Partnering with a friend, a therapist, a support group, a nutritionist, or any number of other personal and professional helpers may make it easier to reach your health goals. Choose your support carefully. You want people on your team who are genuinely interested in your well-being.

14. Your plate is a thing of beauty

If you're eating more fruits and vegetables, your plate is probably bursting with color. Red peppers, leafy greens, deep orange sweet potatoes — colors so bright and bold you may feel compelled to join the millions who photograph their food before diving in.

15. Your wallet doesn't miss the drive-thru

If you're doing more meal prep and less eating out, or if you're eating more whole foods and fewer processed ones, your budget and your body may both be getting healthier.

My NSV's

1.

2.

3.

Rewards

It is the things we work hardest for that will reward us the most.

Often, food was used as a reward. If you had good grades, received an award, or behaved well, parents often used food as a reward. This makes this behavior "normalized" and this pattern can continue into adulthood. Even certain foods can be "love" foods to you. Think about grandma's cooking and smells in the kitchen.

Have you ever looked at your clothes and think "that will never fit!" And then you just slide right in. Learning to reward yourself with non-food activities is the key to success and a lot of fun!

20 Ways to Reward Yourself without Food.
Check all that apply:

☐ Take cooking classes

- ☐ New pretty water bottle
- ☐ Meet with a personal trainer, nutritionist, or health coach
- ☐ New workout clothes
- ☐ A day getaway
- ☐ New candle
- ☐ Take a nap
- ☐ Relaxing massage
- ☐ A gym membership
- ☐ Buy a new cookbook
- ☐ Browse in a bookstore
- ☐ Get a bike
- ☐ Manicure or pedicure
- ☐ Dance classes
- ☐ Professional make up lesson
- ☐ Spa day at home
- ☐ Shop at the Farmer's market
- ☐ Aromatherapy oils
- ☐ Color in an adult coloring book
- ☐ New hair cut

Do you reward yourself with food? Explain.

_____

_____

_____

What non-food ways do you reward yourself?

_____

_____

_____

What non-food ways do you want to try?

_____

_____

_____

Never give up...

Most people don't know your story, your struggles, your hustles, or your prayers. Most people don't know you are fighting and losing some of your silent battles. But here you are, never losing hope. Never give up.

I am proud of you.

— Quotes Café

Positives

"Once you believe in yourself, and you put your mind to something, you can do it."

— Simone Biles

Throughout your bariatric journey there will be many positive things that you will experience. Sometimes it's easier to focus on the negatives than the positives. Make a point to focus on looking for the positives every day. Yes, you will have ups and downs, but you have been given a new life!

Recognize and celebrate all the good things that are happening to you, your health, and your new body. Start a positives journal where you add to it every day. That way when you are feeling down you can go back and read all the positives that have happened to you.

What are some of the positive things that have happened to you?

_____

_____

_____

Which ones have been a total surprise to you?

_____

_____

_____

Gratitude

"Gratitude blocks toxic emotions, such as envy, resentment, regret and depression, which can destroy our happiness."
—Robert Emmons

Do you tend to focus on the negative, things you want, or things you don't have? When you change your thoughts to look and appreciate what you *do* have, your whole perspective changes. This is called gratitude. It involves recognizing and being thankful for what *is* right in your life…in your world. Being thankful and appreciative for what is good instead of looking at what is bad has great mental health benefits. Gratitude is a positive emotion that will cause you to feel an overwhelming source of happiness and positivity.

Start a gratitude journal that you read and add to every day. You should identify and acknowledge the things on your gratitude list. There are many things you can be grateful for. It could be family, other people, achievements, finances, or possessions. As you practice gratitude, it will become easier, more natural, and will become an acquired skill.

Many benefits of gratitude can impact both your mental and physical health. These include:
- Lower your blood pressure
- Have better quality of sleep
- Decrease your stress level
- Have stronger relationships
- Cause less anxiety and depression
- Feel more optimistic
- Increase self-esteem

Ask yourself these questions:
1. Do you have people in your life you are grateful for?
2. Look at where you live - your home, town, state, country. Are there things you can be grateful for?
3. Can you afford the very basics of life - food, shelter and living expenses?

4. Do you have moments of gratitude throughout the day?
5. Can you make a list of people you can turn to if you need help?

Check all A – Z's that you are grateful for:

- ☐ A: Air
- ☐ B: Books
- ☐ C: Coffee
- ☐ D: Dreams
- ☐ E: Electricity
- ☐ F: Family and Friends
- ☐ G: Gifts
- ☐ H: Health
- ☐ I: Internet
- ☐ J: Journaling
- ☐ K: Kindness
- ☐ L: Love and Life
- ☐ M: Memorable Moments
- ☐ N: Nature

- ☐ O: Opportunities
- ☐ P: Pets
- ☐ Q: Quality
- ☐ R: Rest and Relaxation
- ☐ S: Smiles
- ☐ T: Technology
- ☐ U: UtterlyPositive.com
- ☐ V: Victories
- ☐ W: Weekends
- ☐ X: Xmas
- ☐ Y: You
- ☐ Z: Zest

ADD YOUR OWN:

1.

2.

3.

Realizations

"Great things never came from comfort zones."

— Neil Strauss

Positive and negative realizations after bariatric surgery will happen. Some you knew about, and some will be total surprises. Do you feel stronger each day? Do you enjoy changing clothes sizes? Do you have more energy?

Every person will have their own experiences and journeys. Read, listen, and take in what they say. Then formulate your own opinions. Recognize your own realizations.

What realizations have you had since surgery?

_____
_____
_____

Which ones were expected?

_____

_____

_____

Which ones were a surprise?

_____

_____

_____

Chapter 9

Physical Benefits

"When I lost my weight and kept it off, it's when I lost it slowly. I know that expression 'the turtle wins the race'. Now I know that if I lose weight in a healthy way, I keep it off."

— Khloé Kardashian

What some of the bariatric community has said:

1. I may not get to goal weight.
2. The less you have to lose, the slower the loss.
3. I may not be able to stop losing weight.
4. People will watch and criticize what I eat.
5. There's a high when losing and a low when you stall.
6. It's normal to go up and down a few pounds.
7. Most of the weight comes off in the first year.

8. Being so terrified/obsessed with gaining weight back.
9. Don't weigh daily.
10. Stalls are normal.
11. I know that even with stalls I can continue this and not give up.
12. We lost weight and we are looking good.
13. Feet can shrink sizes.
14. Would look older and have more wrinkles
15. How awesome I'd look and feel.
16. Would look younger.
17. Would look older and have more wrinkles.
18. You might look younger or older.
19. Feels good to actually reach an itch on my back…It's the little things.
20. Remember that we all have different bodies, weights, and goals. Don't get discouraged if you see other results and yours is different.
21. Diabetes would not go away right away after surgery.
22. Almost all my co-morbidities would go away.

23. How tired I'd be for a few months.

24. How quickly my health has improved.

25. In the beginning I'd be very tired.

26. The journey would add years to your life.

27. That my gallbladder would need to be removed.

28. Care for my teeth better.

Weight Loss

Losing weight is hard. Being overweight is hard. Choose your hard.

During your weight loss journey, there will be many peaks and valleys. Remember, it's not a race, it's a marathon. Longevity is the *key* to success. If you follow the rules, you *will* lose weight. Continuing to live by the rules will ensure you will keep the weight off. This is a necessity for living in wellness.

Not only will you lose weight, but there will also be many non-scale victories (NSV's). Learn to recognize and celebrate them. Other bariatric patients have reported not only losses in their body, but in their fingers (ring sizes), feet (shoe sizes), face (glasses), and head (hat sizes). Shoes fall off, underwear falls down and bras don't fit anymore. It's amazing to see all the changes that happen to your body.

Remember if you're losing slow, the weight didn't come on all at once. You will stall. Trust the process. Go to the gym or outside and just walk. If your body is starving, your metabolism will slow down. Starvation mode creates a hormone imbalance that causes your body to store fat. If your body thinks it will get fed regularly, it actually slows down and burns calories.

You can't always believe the scale. Try on clothes you haven't worn in a while. Sometimes weight loss is in inches not weight. Sometimes losing weight in your middle area, hips, or thighs is the last to go. Usually, whatever body parts you hold the most weight in are the slowest to lose.

Tips to Know:

- Slower is better.
- It's not always about the number on the scale.
- Weight loss can vary from week to week.
- Weight loss is not immediate.
- Eating less is not always the answer.
- The goal is to lose fat, not just weight.

Check all that apply:

- ☐ Analyze your food intake to determine if you need an adjustment
- ☐ Acknowledge inches along with weight loss
- ☐ Move more
- ☐ Get better sleep
- ☐ Eat slower
- ☐ Get outside and walk
- ☐ Drink more water
- ☐ Meet your protein goals
- ☐ Recognize the NSV's

Looks Change

"It's so important for women to look the way they want to look and feel the way they want to feel for their own reasons, not because someone's telling them to or because it's fashionable or trendy."

— Kirstie Alley

It only takes one day to decide you *are* enough and do something positive about it. It takes a few weeks to notice your weight loss and possibly longer for your friends and the world to notice. But you will be the first one to notice as the changes happen. There will obviously be weight loss but many non-scale victories too.

Sometimes when your looks change it will be hard for you to accept the changes. This is only because they are not familiar. What *is* familiar is the bigger you. Notice the subtle changes as they happen. Usually, the bigger places on your body will be the last places to lose. Don't let that discourage you. The weight will come off.

Take lots of pictures so you can compare the before and after. Keep trying on a goal outfit, even if it's one size smaller than where you started. Measure yourself. Many times, inches will come off before pounds.

When your looks change, people will notice. Those that didn't pay any attention to you may suddenly compliment or look at you differently. This can be uncomfortable especially if it is from the opposite sex. Attention can be hard or even make you angry. "If you didn't like me before, why are you liking me now?"

Fat shaming people is real. It's more of *their* problem and not *yours*. You will become more attractive and even dress nicer. People of the same sex may become jealous and treat you differently. This can include your friends. It can be okay for you to lose weight, but just not *too* much weight. And low and behold, don't get any thinner than them. If you have always being the heavier one in the group, it will be hard for them as that role shifts. Again, remember it's *their* problem not *yours*. Just be prepared.

Where did you notice the first place you lost weight?

_____

_____

_____

How far along were you?

_____

_____

_____

Who noticed your weight loss first? What did they say?

_____

_____

_____

Who is having a hard time with your looks changing?

_____

_____

_____

Health

"Fitness: If it came in a bottle, everybody would have a great body."

— Cher

With bariatric surgery, your health will improve. That's a given. How soon or what health problems will improve is not something you can predict or control. Somethings about your health will get better immediately. Your doctor may even discontinue some of your medications at the time of your surgery.

Right after surgery you will be tired and in pain. Your body is adjusting and healing from major surgery. This will improve and pass. Just be patient with yourself and let your body heal and recover. Don't rush any of the processes, especially the stages of food. Also, it's very important to eat according to your plan. Your new stomach is healing, and you wouldn't want to risk damaging it.

Bariatric surgery does not come without risks. Know this going in. Some people need to have their gall bladder removed while others do not. Also, acid reflux can happen. People can dump when eating something too sweet. Depending on the type of surgery you have, there may be other risks associated with the surgery.

Be sure to take all your required vitamins and minerals daily to have optimal health. Overall, your physical health will improve. You will have more energy and be able to enjoy the things you couldn't do before surgery. Embrace the changes and the new you!

What health problems or co-morbidities do you have?

_____

_____

_____

What medications do you take daily?

_____

_____

_____

What medications did your doctor take you off of immediately?

_____

_____

_____

What health conditions has your doctor said will go away?

_____

_____

_____

Chapter 10

Struggles

"Strength and growth come only through continuous effort and struggle".

— Napoleon Hill

What some of the bariatric community has said:

1. I'm having a hard time with the food.
2. Some days I wonder if this is as good as it gets.
3. I worry about the long-term effects of the surgery.
4. I hate myself that I've had to go to these drastic ways to lose weight.
5. Why couldn't I do it on my own?
6. My appetite would return to normal.
7. Nothing looks good or sounds good to eat.
8. Every meal I eat past the one bite that says "enough," I suffer for it.

9. Acid reflux can happen.
10. Complications can happen to anyone.
11. Dumping syndrome is very painful.
12. Malnutrition can happen.
13. Stomach rumbling and sneezing or hiccups when full.
14. Listen to that first sign of being full.
15. Burp or hiccup when full
16. Always freezing.
17. Reflux is a complication for many.
18. The hair loss was so bad.
19. Your electrolytes and potassium levels can go out of balance.
20. Hormones can get out of wack with rapid weight loss.
21. Dehydration will happen if not drinking enough fluids.
22. Miss my extra padding on my butt.
23. Dumping causes foamies.
24. I'd have a sore tailbone.
25. Bat wings are from losing arm fat.

26. My neck looks like a turkey.
27. Stalls are normal. Starvation is not.
28. Dizziness/Light-headedness can happen when not well hydrated.
29. Pay attention to restriction.
30. My nose runs uncontrollably.
31. Body itching can happen after surgery.
32. Joints and back hurting from losing cushion.
33. How my knees and hips hurt from the weight loss.
34. Body aches from losing fat so fast.
35. Constant struggle with constipation or diarrhea.
36. Will need to take stool softeners and laxatives all the time.
37. Constipation is horrible.
38. Constant stinky gas.
39. Smelly gas.
40. Constipation is a real thing.
41. You will feel bones you never felt before.
42. Knee bones will hurt when laying on your side.

43. Hips and knees will hurt from the shifting weight loss.
44. I can feel hip bones even though I never did.
45. My rib bones stick out.
46. I didn't know what my breastbone was before.
47. I don't like having collarbones.
48. Just how much harder it would be.
49. Was sad and crying for a time.
50. Wishing I had a different surgery.
51. That I would no longer enjoy food.
52. Hitting a rough patch doesn't undo the progress you've made.
53. Whenever you find yourself doubting how far you can go, just remember how far you have come.
54. I should have gotten therapy before the surgery. Food was my medicine.
55. I miss eating with my family.
56. I have no energy.
57. I need to learn how to stay motivated.
58. I wish I had the gastric bypass.

59. The journey has been so hard.
60. Other people have done better than me. I must be doing something wrong.
61. You might get more wrinkles.
62. Start saving money ASAP for extra skin removal.
63. Skin will sag.
64. I have creepy skin on my arms and legs.
65. The slower the better for your skin elasticity and plenty of water.
66. Moisturizing skin is so important.
67. Age plays a factor in skin's elasticity.
68. The doctor took 9 lbs. of extra skin off.
69. Post-op puking is no fun.
70. You will regret it once it happens to you.
71. It's the worst feeling ever.
72. Once it happens to you, you get it.
73. Some foods make me dump once but not again.
74. Regain isn't a matter of IF, it's a matter of WHEN if I don't follow the rules.
75. Set a hard gain limit.

76. It would be easy to overeat and regain.
77. Don't think that a bite here or there won't hurt you.
78. Regain and relapse can happen.
79. Regain weight is harder to lose than surgery weight.
80. I do not eat anything off plan, but I do "graze" and eat too much at times of the healthy food.
81. Fact is, too many calories = regain.
82. I've had a lot going on and as much as I would love to blame, but the fact is, the choices were mine.
83. I've fallen off the wagon!
84. Help! I've gained weight again and I don't know why...
85. All my old habits are starting to creep back in and I don't know what to do!
86. I think I stretched out my pouch.
87. I knew I'd be a failure.

Struggles

Where there is no struggle, there is no progress.

Struggles are part of having bariatric surgery. Besides physical struggles with the surgery itself, you will have mental and emotional struggles too. Some days you will doubt, regret, and question your decision to have surgery. You will wonder why you couldn't do it on your own and may feel shame. You will forget the reasons you chose in the first place.

Feelings of anger, frustration, and even depression can overtake you. If you've had to pay for the surgery, the added financial pressure can mount. Maybe you've had to save a long time or even had to get a loan. Thoughts can creep in like was the surgery even worth it after you have paid so much to have it.

People looking for weight loss surgery have a history of fat shaming, bullying, low self-esteem and difficulties in dating that can contribute to depression. You may also experience shame and hopelessness because the diets and exercise routines you tried didn't work. As for binge eating, it is often a method of using food to cope with negative emotions rather than expressing them or finding a healthy treatment such as psychotherapy (Rauch, 2016).

There are many stages you will go through. Talk to others who have already had bariatric surgery. Seek counseling if it becomes more than you can handle.

What emotional stages have you gone through?
_____
_____
_____

What regrets do you have?
_____
_____
_____

What struggles do you have?
_____
_____
_____

Body Side Effects

"If you take care of your body, it'll take care of you."
— Usher

Learn the signs when your body is full. Sometimes your stomach will growl and gurgle. You may burp, sneeze or hiccup. That is the time to stop. It's your body's alarm clock. If you learn these signs early on, you won't overeat.

It's a hard adjustment to still see food left on your plate. It's better to serve yourself less food, that way you won't feel guilty for throwing uneaten food away. Plus, if you continue to eat past full, you will be in pain and probably throw up.

Trust your bariatric doctor. They have evaluated your health issues and determined if you would be a great candidate for bariatric surgery. The benefits can outweigh the risks.

As your body weight changes there will be some side effects. Arms develop "bat wings." Your butt will be flat, and your tailbone will hurt. These changes are part of the bariatric life process. You will adapt and learn. Your new life will become more comfortable than your old life and you will grow to *love* the new you and new body.

What side effects have you had?
_____
_____
_____

What have you done about these side effects?
_____
_____
_____

Pain

"Pain is inevitable, suffering is optional."

— Buddha

After your bariatric surgery you will have pain. You've just had major surgery and your body will hurt. How long you will hurt depends on a lot of factors. If you've had complications during the surgery or recovery, you will have more or longer pain. Don't suffer alone. Speak to your doctor if you're having unusual or prolonged pain.

During your new journey you may have pain. Learn what is normal pain and abnormal pain. Do not rely on the advice of your friends or family. Speak to your doctor. Often it is temporary stages your body goes through. It will get better. All pain should be explainable. No one should be in lasting pain.

In the beginning of an exercise routine, you will have pain. As you stretch and work the muscles, you will hurt. But in time this will get better and you will be stronger. Muscle replaces fat, so that's a good thing.

Mental pain is another whole issue. Many adjustments to your new life take time. It is best to address any emotional or mental issues *before* surgery. Bariatric life will be completely different than the life you had before. Always remember the reasons you chose to have the surgery.

Many months of preparation have been done to prepare you. But sometimes until you actually have the surgery does the head catch up to the body. This means that even if you have the knowledge before surgery, when you're actually living it, it will become your new reality. Don't hesitate to seek counseling if you feel like it is too much to handle on your own.

Bowels

"The best thing is to realize that you are who you are and you gotta work with what you got."

— Zendaya

Gas

During your bariatric surgery, you will be filled with gas to make it easier for your surgeon to navigate inside your body. After surgery, movement will ease the gas pains and help it to go away.

You need to move and walk it off. Take as many trips in the hallway as you can when you are recovering from surgery. Once home, you will need to continue walking. Pain in your shoulder is common after surgery from the gas.

Many people report having stinky gas during healing. Your body is healing, and your digestion is changing. This may last for awhile or even permanently. It's just part of the process.

Constipation

A very common side effect of bariatric surgery is constipation and can become very painful. Have medication on hand to help with constipation. Don't wait too long before taking medication. You can easily get blocked up. This is even *more* painful than just constipation. If not relieved, it may require you to go to the hospital ER where they can unblock your colon.

Diarrhea

Diarrhea can be *very* dangerous as your electrolytes can get out of balance. It can also cause arrhythmias and fainting. You may need IV hydrations and stool medication. You need to contact your doctor as soon as possible.

Living with diarrhea can also be a side effect of your medication. Have your doctor look at everything you are on to decide if a change in medication is needed. For explosive or sudden diarrhea, you should always carry a change of clothes and some wipes. Better to be prepared than be caught off guard.

Bones

"Our bodies change. Our minds change. Our hearts change."

— Emma Stone

As someone who may have been overweight most of your life, you may have never felt certain bones in your body before. When you start dropping weight, bones will be more noticeable, either by sight or feel. This can take some getting used to. Your body can hurt in your hips or knees as your weight shifts. This will level off and is temporary.

Some sleeping positions may become uncomfortable. Laying on your side, knee bone to knee bone can hurt. Learn to shift positions. Perhaps slide one leg slightly lower that the other.

A lot of people also complain about feeling bones in their butt when sitting in a chair. If it's an office chair, get a cushion to use. Building muscle will also help with feeling pain from bones after losing weight and muscle.

Collar bones will be new to you. At first, it may seem weird or strange. You may not even like the way they look or feel. But you will get there. Look at other thin people or celebrities and notice that they all have beautiful collar bones. Emotionally it might take a while to get used to seeing and feeling your bones. Embrace it, make peace with it. It's the new healthier, you!

What bones have you felt first? Second? Third?

_____

_____

_____

Regrets

"Don't be afraid of failure, this is the way to succeed."
— Lebron James

Part of the recovery process is regrets. Especially the first few days after your surgery. Regrets are normal! This stage is temporary. For people that have never had major surgery, the pain you will be in may be enough for you to question your decision to have the surgery. This too *will* pass. Give it time and be patient. Remember the reasons you chose to have bariatric surgery.

Any number of other things can make you fall into regret. If you're not losing weight fast enough may cause regret. At this time, evaluate what you're eating. Stalls are normal and part of the process.

Sometimes you may wonder if you should have gotten a different bariatric surgery, especially if you're having problems now. When you compare yourself to others who had a different surgery than you, you may begin to question if you made the right decision. Many people do have another bariatric surgery after the first one. For example, going from having a lap band to another type of bariatric surgery is common. Also, going from having a gastric sleeve to gastric bypass is something people choose.

Food may have a different taste to you now. Foods that you enjoyed before may not taste well or sit well in your new pouch. This can be upsetting or even depressing. Try these foods at different times as your taste buds do change.

Address all your mental and emotional issues *first*. You will have emotional changes and adjustments after surgery. It is better to have a jump start on the mental part before surgery. If you need additional help after surgery, seek out a professional therapist.

10 Regrets from other Bariatric Patients: (Mexicobariatriccenter, 2023)

1. I regret not getting it sooner…
2. It's a lot of work

3. I regret not having realistic expectations
4. I regret not having gastric bypass surgery (instead of the gastric sleeve)
5. I regret not knowing how much my relationship with food would change
6. Hair Loss. I regret not being able to avoid hair loss
7. Body Dysmorphia: being mentally and emotionally prepared
8. Excess skin is difficult to manage after losing weight
9. I regret not learning how to eat slowly before surgery
10. Not being able to enjoy food

What regrets do you have?

_____

_____

_____

Burnout

"If you're trying to achieve, there will be roadblocks. I've had them, everybody has had them. But obstacles don't have to stop you. If you run into a wall, don't turn around and give up. Figure out how to climb it, go through it, or work around it."

— Michael Jordan

A combination of mental, physical, and emotional stress can cause burnout. Are you tired of following your food plan? Do you hate exercise? Is it hard for you to recognize the new you? You can be feeling burnout. But not all is lost. The good news is that there *are* ways to combat burnout.

Add meaning to your daily activities. If you lack meaning in your life, you can feel burnout. Look at the big picture in your day. Are you doing something good for yourself? Are you helping others? Are you taking care of your pets? Find something meaningful for the day to do.

Look for gratitude. Make a gratitude list and focus on all what you are grateful for in your life. Sometimes focusing on the negative can cause burn out. Add something new each day to your gratitude list. Read over your list once a day in the morning or at night before bed.

Choose stress-reducing activities. Adding an activity to your daily routine can be very helpful to fight burnout. What are you doing to reduce stress? Do you garden? Go to the gym? Walk around the neighborhood? Do you have friends or family you can talk to when you need to vent?

Check all that you do for burnout:
- ☐ Scrapbooking
- ☐ Reading
- ☐ Puzzles
- ☐ Yoga
- ☐ Photography
- ☐ Swimming

- ☐ Knitting
- ☐ Baking
- ☐ Carving
- ☐ Walking a pet
- ☐ Play cards
- ☐ Pottery
- ☐ Hiking
- ☐ Scuba diving
- ☐ Painting
- ☐ Beach combing
- ☐ Cross stitch
- ☐ Computer games
- ☐ Social media
- ☐ Fishing
- ☐ Gardening
- ☐ Tennis
- ☐ Coloring
- ☐ Camping
- ☐ Music

ADD YOUR OWN:

1.

2.

3.

4.

5.

Skin

Remember: Bariatric surgery is a medical surgery, not a cosmetic one!

Bariatric surgery is an excellent option for significant weight loss. Whenever massive weight loss occurs, especially in a short amount of time, loose skin is inevitable. The skin doesn't have the ability to tighten up as quickly and easily. This is a normal and expected outcome. The greater the weight loss after bariatric surgery generally results in more excess skin. This can cause discomfort too.

Loose skin can be more of a nuisance than a problem. Some issues that can arise with loose skin aside from appearance, include chafing, irritation, rashes, and discomfort. It can also carry risks of infection. These risks can be managed by preventing friction and skin to skin contact by wearing compression clothing, applying loose powder, or using baby diaper rash ointment in between layers of excess skin.

Compression clothing holds your skin in place and prevents rubbing, which can eliminate discomfort. In rare cases, loose skin after weight loss surgery impairs a person's ability to be physically active. Common places to notice excess skin include the abdomen, buttocks, and upper arms.

Factors that Affect the Elasticity of the Skin

A variety of factors exist that can affect skin elasticity - age, amount of weight lost, nutrition, genetics, and smoking status. Certain medical conditions can also impact the thinning of your skin and determine how well your skin is able to adapt to major weight loss. While some of these factors are controllable, some are out of your control.

Controllable Factors

Diet

Exercise

Weight Maintenance

    Hydration

    Supplements

    Cosmetic surgery

Un-controllable Factors

    Age

    Genetics

    Pre-existing Medical Conditions

How do you feel about having excess and loose skin?

_____

_____

_____

Have you considered cosmetic surgery for skin removal? Why or why not?

_____

_____

_____

Losing too much Weight

Never let a stumble in the road be the end of the journey.

What some of the bariatric community has said:
1. Eat some high fiber carbs, healthy oils, and healthy treats.
2. Eat more calories and protein.
3. Don't worry it will slow down and you may even stall.
4. Ask your dietician and doctor for advice.
5. Check your medicines.

Who would have thought losing too much weight could be a problem for you? After being overweight for so long your initial thought may have been, "Yes, I'd love to have that problem." But losing too much weight can be a problem if you become malnourished or sick. Others will see it before you will. Many times, when you are looking good, people will tell you that you need to stop losing weight. That can be just an adjustment on their part as they are used to seeing you overweight. Always consult with your doctor.

If you added carbs and some other less healthier foods and you're still losing weight, check with your doctor. It could be that you aren't getting in enough calories which then causes the body to go into starvation mode. The body will react much differently if it thinks you are starving it.

Add in exercise. Build muscle. This can help your weight sustain. Make exercise a part of your everyday routine. Overall, you will feel better too.

Check your medicine with your doctor. Often there are medicines that you take for one thing and a side effect can be losing weight. Discuss the pros and cons.

Look at an ideal weight chart. Maybe since you have always been overweight you may not ever thought of yourself as being able to get this thin. You may be at a normal weight for your height. Try to stay off the scale. Use your clothes as a good judgement. Just because you've never been this weight before doesn't mean that it's not a good weight for your body.

When was the last time you were this weight?

_____
_____
_____

How does it feel to be this weight?

_____
_____
_____

Grazing

You can't be doing the same thing over and over again expecting different results.

Grazing is the repetitive eating of small amounts of food in an unplanned manner throughout the day. It is *not* in response to hunger. It can be compulsive or non-compulsive eating. Grazing happens when you snack all day on slider foods. Slider foods are anything that can "slide" down easily. With having no volume to them, they are usually higher in calories. It is easy to mindlessly eat them especially when doing other things like watching TV, working on the computer, or talking on the phone.

Can grazing ever be a good thing? Yes, grazing on healthy snacks can level off blood sugar. It becomes a bad idea when you snack on unhealthy foods such as grab and go types of food. Think about sitting and eating out of a bag of chips. It's a mindless act and before you know it you've eaten way more than you should.

What foods do you graze on?

_____

_____

_____

What foods do you need to eliminate from your house?

_____

_____

_____

Dumping

Aim for progress over perfection.

Dumping happens when you overeat, need to throw up and only "foam" comes up. Some people refer to it as "bubbly saliva." It is unpleasant at best. This can happen if a food you eat doesn't agree with you too. Too much sugar can make you dump. Your body will let you know when it rejects something you ate.

You feel like you're going to projectile vomit, only a liquid foam comes up. You must sit with this feeling until it passes. Dumping causes you to overall feel awful. You will learn not to eat certain foods again or overeat after experiencing dumping. Gastric bypass patients tend to experience dumping more than other types of bariatric surgery. Dumping is not fun!!

Two types of dumping include immediate dumping and late dumping. Immediate dumping happens right after you eat. Physically you can get a horrible pain or cramps, sweats, shaking, bloating, nausea, vomiting, diarrhea, flushing, chills, dizziness, lightheadedness, or rapid heartbeat. Late dumping happens 1 - 3 hours after you eat a high sugar meal. Physically you can get low blood sugar from the pancreas releasing too much insulin, sweating, flushing, chills, dizziness, lightheadedness, weakness, or rapid heartbeat.

What foods have caused you to dump?

_____
_____
_____

What dumping symptoms have you had?

_____
_____
_____

Regain

"Do not be embarrassed by your failures, learn from them and start again."

— Richard Branson

Struggling with weight regain? Do you feel like a failure? Try not to beat yourself up or feel guilty. That might be easier said than done. Beating yourself up about being a "failure" will make things worse, especially if you tend to turn to food for emotional comfort. If you are off track, you need to reset your mind and body to restart weight loss. Remember, a bariatric journey requires *consistent* effort if you want to maintain the results of your bariatric surgery.

Instead of dwelling on the past or the negatives, think about all the success you have achieved so far, where you've come from, the positive things you've gained and the habits you have kept since your surgery. Then, think about what you might need to adjust to move forward. Your bariatric life is a *lifetime* journey. For some, a bit of weight regain is part of that journey. Getting back on track with your new habits is the next step of the process. If you feel like your mindset is holding you back, consider speaking with a therapist.

It's important to dust off your knees and go on when you fall, not stay stuck in the dirt. Don't be discouraged, you are *not* alone. When the "honeymoon" period comes to an end, some of your weight can sneak back on. The good news is that there is always something that can be done. Restarting weight loss is definitely achievable, provided you maintain a healthy lifestyle change. This will get you back on the path to long-term success.

Regain is real and will happen if you decide to abandon the rules. Give yourself a weight window such as 5 lbs. It is ok if you fluctuate by this amount, but if you go one pound over, then tighten up your food and/or exercise. Weight fluctuation is *normal*. It is advisable to only weigh once a week. Don't let the scale dictate your success. Often you will lose inches instead of pounds. If you are exercising, you will be building muscle which weighs more. Keep doing what you're doing and don't get discouraged.

Evaluate your Daily Routine:

Are you eating too quickly?
1. Take small bites, use small utensils, and one piece of food at a time.
2. Chew until nothing is left and then swallow.
3. Take another bite after you have completely chewed and swallowed the previous bite.

Are you choosing foods not on your plan?
1. Plan your meals ahead of time.
2. Don't go to the grocery hungry.
3. Focus just on today and today's meals.

Are you grazing?
1. Remove easily grazing foods from your house like nuts or chips.

2. Before you grab something, ask yourself if you're hungry or just grabbing food out of habit.
3. Stick to all planned snacks and meals.

Are you getting enough water?
1. Sometimes when you think you are hungry, you are just thirsty.
2. Drinking enough water in a day keeps you hydrated and less hungry.
3. Add flavor packets to your water to make them tastier.

Are you eating protein first and enough protein in a day?
1. You want to fill up on protein first to stay full longer.
2. Focus on protein rich foods.
3. Eat a variety of protein options to prevent boredom.

In what ways have you slipped back into old habits/foods?

_____

_____

_____

What can you tighten up in your daily routine?

_____

_____

_____

Back to Basics

"Start where you are. Use what you have. Do what you can."

— Arthur Ashe

Usually when people have regained some weight, they have started eating like they did before their surgery. Perhaps your portion sizes have increased? Maybe your food choices have become careless? Could it be the quality of your meals causing you to not stay full very long? Are you grazing? Have you dropped the rules that must be followed? If any of these sound like you, go back to the basics and look at *how* you're eating (slow down, be mindful). Check in with your appetite and ask if you're hungry or if you're eating for other reasons.

A bariatric pouch reset diet is like your post-surgery diet that lasted for 8-10 weeks. Fortunately, the reset typically lasts only 1-2 weeks. However, since you'll be drastically limiting your food intake, it's crucial that you follow up with your surgeon and registered dietitian during a bariatric pouch reset.

Weight fluctuations *happen*...you might not be eating enough or might be eating too much of the wrong thing. Tighten up your regime and eliminate extras.

Start tracking everything you eat by documenting all food and water intake. Using an app on your phone can be very helpful as it causes you to be disciplined and consistent. See where you can adjust.

Stay away from empty carbs like white potatoes, bread, rice, and pasta. Limit or eliminate other carbs to get back on track. Avoid all high fat food. Get to your goal weight and then you can reincorporate healthy carbs.

Stop grazing and remove all grazing foods such as nuts and chips from your sight. Grazing foods can be a mindless eating activity. Remember the rules. High protein, low carbs, extremely low sugar at every meal and every snack. Protein first, healthy veggies after. Eat anything protein packed. Increase your water intake. Spend some time focusing only on protein and water goals.

You may lose a few pounds being on a liquid diet, but you're highly likely to regain all of it when you're back on a regular diet again unless you change your mindset. Get back to basics even if starting over can feel intimidating. You need to refocus. If you stay consistent and work hard, you can get back on track and lose the extra weight you may have gained back.

Check all that you do:

- ☐ Ask yourself if you're hungry before you eat
- ☐ Eat only when you're hungry
- ☐ Eat protein at each meal and snack
- ☐ Eat (at least at lunch and dinner) a meal that is half protein and half veg
- ☐ Eat a variety of foods throughout the day/week
- ☐ Take 20-30 minutes to eat your meal
- ☐ Take teaspoon-sized mouthfuls

- ☐ Concentrate on your meals while eating
- ☐ Don't eat in front of the TV or computer or in the car
- ☐ Choose calorie-free fluids during the day
- ☐ Drink at least 1.5L of fluid per day
- ☐ Take your supplements each day
- ☐ Move throughout the day
- ☐ Take some time each day for yourself

SCALE

Why do I allow you to control me?

You tell me if I've done good or bad.

You even make me like or hate myself.

I must let you go.

You have no power over me…anymore!

— Anonymous

Part III -

BONUS: What I am looking forward to after weight loss

Check all that apply:

- ☐ Acknowledging that "I did it"
- ☐ Be healthier
- ☐ Be in family photos
- ☐ Bend over
- ☐ Cut my toenails and breathe at the same time
- ☐ Cross my legs
- ☐ Eat salad and enjoy it
- ☐ Enjoy sex more
- ☐ Exercise is easier
- ☐ Feel beautiful
- ☐ Feel comfortable in my own skin
- ☐ Feel good in my body
- ☐ Fit in an airplane seat
- ☐ Fit into "cute" clothes
- ☐ Fit into smaller clothes
- ☐ Fly comfortably
- ☐ Get better sleep
- ☐ Get off medications
- ☐ Get out of a tub easily

- ☐ Get out of my wheelchair
- ☐ Get rid of my fat clothes
- ☐ Get toned
- ☐ Get my basic hygiene back
- ☐ Get rid of my CPAP machine
- ☐ Go tubing
- ☐ Have a child sit on my lap
- ☐ Have ankles again
- ☐ Have less co-morbidities
- ☐ Have less pain
- ☐ Have more energy
- ☐ Have more stamina
- ☐ Have only 1 or 2 sizes in my closet
- ☐ Have someone call me "skinny"
- ☐ Have way more energy
- ☐ Hike
- ☐ Horseback ride
- ☐ I want to choose life
- ☐ Jog/run
- ☐ Kayak
- ☐ Keep up with the grandkids

- ☐ Like what I see in a mirror or building window reflection
- ☐ Live longer
- ☐ Live my best life
- ☐ Look better and feel better
- ☐ Look down and see my toes
- ☐ Marathon
- ☐ Mountain biking
- ☐ No fear of breaking chairs when sitting
- ☐ No longer feeling like the "fat friend"
- ☐ No more plus-sized clothes
- ☐ No more snoring
- ☐ Not always be the photographer
- ☐ No thighs rubbing
- ☐ Not need a bra extension
- ☐ Not need a seatbelt extension
- ☐ Paddleboard
- ☐ Put on socks
- ☐ Realize that you look normal now
- ☐ Reduce chances for heart attack/stroke
- ☐ Reduced joint pain

- ☐ Reduce medications
- ☐ Ride a mule down a mountain
- ☐ Ride amusement park rides
- ☐ Ride a bike
- ☐ Ride a motorcycle
- ☐ Reach and wipe my butt
- ☐ Rock climb
- ☐ See people's reactions
- ☐ Set a healthy example for my kids
- ☐ Shave my legs
- ☐ Shop in regular sized sections
- ☐ Show up
- ☐ Sit and bathe in a tub
- ☐ Sit on the floor
- ☐ Skate
- ☐ Ski
- ☐ Skydive
- ☐ Stomach not hitting the steering wheel
- ☐ Sweat less
- ☐ Swim
- ☐ Tie my shoes

- ☐ To hear, "You are at goal weight"
- ☐ Travel more
- ☐ Tuck my shirt in
- ☐ Wakeboarding
- ☐ Walk into a clothes shop and buy a smaller size off the rack
- ☐ Walk more
- ☐ Walk up and down stairs
- ☐ Walk without a device
- ☐ Walk without my legs rubbing together
- ☐ Walk without pain
- ☐ Water ski
- ☐ Wear a belt
- ☐ Wear a bikini
- ☐ Wear a swimsuit and not feel self-conscience
- ☐ Wear boots
- ☐ Wear cute undergarments
- ☐ Wear designer brands
- ☐ Wear form-fitting clothes
- ☐ Wear non-stretchy clothes
- ☐ Wear shoes with ankle straps

- ☐ Wear my "some day" clothes in the back of the closet
- ☐ Wear shorts in public
- ☐ Wear zip-up jeans
- ☐ Whitewater rafting
- ☐ Zipline

ADD YOUR OWN:

1.

2.

3.

4.

5.

References

Ackerman, C. (2018, May 23). *22 Examples of High Self-Esteem*. Positivepsychology.com. Retrieved July 19, 2023, from https://positivepsychology.com/self-esteem/#examples-self-esteem

Anxiety disorders. Mayoclinic.org. Retrieved July 21, 2023, from
> *https://www.mayoclinic.org/diseases-conditions/anxiety/symptoms-causes/syc-20350961*

A to Z Gratitude List: Letters A-Z. Utterlypositive.com. Retrieved June 7, 2023, from
> https://utterlypositive.com/a-to-z-gratitude-list-alphabet/

Awakening Peace, Inc. (2021). *Awaken your Peace.* Retrieved from
> https://awakeningpeace.org/programs/#awakening

Bariatric surgery. Mayoclinic.org. Retrieved June 4, 2023, from
> https://www.mayoclinic.org/tests-procedures/bariatric-surgery/about/pac-20394258

Body Dysmorphic Disorder (BDD). Clevelandclinic.org. Retrieved July 7, 2023, from
    https://my.clevelandclinic.org/health/diseases/9888-body-dysmorphic-disorder

Body Image. Psychologytoday.com. Retrieved July 13, 2023, from
    https://www.psychologytoday.com/us/basics/body-image

Brabaw, K. (2019, June 10). *Do You Have a Healthy Relationship With Food?* Prevention. Retrieved December 2, 2021, from
    https://www.prevention.com/food-nutrition/a20495831/do-you-have-a-healthy-relationship-with-food/

Canadian Mental Health Association, BC Division (nd). *Body image, self-esteem, and mental health.* Retrieved December 2, 2021, from
    https://www.heretohelp.bc.ca/infosheet/body-image-self-esteem-and-mentalhealth

Cleveland Clinic (2021). *Stress.* Retrieved from
    https://my.clevelandclinic.org/health/articles/11874-stress

Depression (major depressive disorder.) Mayoclinic.org. Retrieved July 21, 2023, from,
    https://www.mayoclinic.org/diseases-

conditions/depression/symptoms-causes/syc-20356007?p=1

Depression. Nimh.nih.gov. Retrieved July 24, 2023, from,
https://www.nimh.nih.gov/health/topics/depression

Effective Coping Skills Used in Eating Disorder Recovery. Retrieved July 13, 2023, from
https://www.eatingdisorderhope.com/recovery/self-help-tools-skills-tips/effective-coping-for-eating-disorders

Exercise after Bariatric Surgery. Sutterhealth.org. Retrieved June 4, 2023, from
https://www.sutterhealth.org/services/weight-loss/exercise-after-bariatricsurgery

Exercise benefits for Bariatric Patients. Sutterhealth.org. Retrieved June 4, 2023, from
https://www.mayoclinichealthsystem.org/hometown-health/speaking-of-health/exercise-benefits-for-bariatric-patients

Gager, E. (nd). *Tips to manage stress eating.* John Hopkins Medicine. Retrieved December 2, 2021, from
https://www.hopkinsmedicine.org/health/wellness-and-prevention/tips-to-manage-stress-eating

Getting started with Mindfulness. Mindful.org. Retrieved May 23, 2023, from
https://www.mindful.org/meditation/mindfulness-getting-started/

Grounding Techniques. Therapistaid.com. Retrieved May 24, 2023, from
https://www.therapistaid.com/worksheets/grounding-techniques

Five strategies for overcoming emotional eating. Psychologytoday.com Retrieved July 19, 2023 from
https://www.psychologytoday.com/us/blog/shrink/201206/five-strategies-overcoming-emotional-eating

5 Ways to Fight Excess Skin after Bariatric Surgery. health.clevelandclinic.org. Retrieved May 25, 2023, from https://health.clevelandclinic.org/5-ways-to-fight-excess-skin-after-your-bariatric-surgery/

Hickey, S-A. (nd). *Emotional eating quiz.* www.health-and-natural-healing.com. Retrieved December 2, 2021, from
https://www.bodytypology.com/emotional-eating-quiz.html

How to Deal with Loose Skin after Weight Loss Surgery. Barilife.com. Retrieved May 25, 2023, from https://www.barilife.com/blog/loose-skin-after-weight-loss-surgery/

How to Restart Weight Loss after Gastric Bypass. Bariatricfusion.com. Retrieved June 4, 2023, from https://www.bariatricfusion.com/blogs/blog/how-to-restart-weight-loss-after-gastric-bypass

Mindfulness exercises. Mayoclinic.org. Retrieved May 23, 2023, from
https://www.mayoclinic.org/healthy-lifestyle/consumer-health/in-depth/mindfulness- exercises/art-20046356

Rauch, J. (2016, November 17). *The Mental Health Struggles of Weight Loss Surgery.* Psychologytoday.com. Retrieved July 26, 2023, from https://www.psychologytoday.com/us/blog/the-truth-about-exercise-addiction/201611/the-mental-health-struggles-weight-loss-surgery

Seitz, A. (2022, May 18). *6 Common Types of Eating Disorders (and their Symptoms).* Healthline.com. Retrieved July 20, 2023, from
https://www.healthline.com/nutrition/common-eating-disorders

Should I take vitamins and supplements after weight loss surgery. Mayoclinic.org. Retrieved May 23, 2023, from https://www.mayoclinichealthsystem.org/hometown-health/speaking-of-health/should-i-take-vitamins-and-supplements-after-weight-loss-surgery

Simple steps to get back on track after sleeve gastrectomy. Livingwithasleeve.com. Retrieved June 4, 2023, from
https://www.livingwithasleeve.com/simple-steps-to-get-back-on-track-after-sleeve-gastrectomy/

Sinrich, J. (nd). *How to stop rewarding yourself with food – AAPTIV.* Retrieved December 2, 2021, from
https://aaptiv.com/magazine/rewarding-yourself-with-food

Sleeve Gastrectomy. Mayoclinic.org. Retrieved June 1, 2023, from
https://www.mayoclinic.org/tests-procedures/sleeve-gastrectomy/about/pac-20385183

Smith, M., Robinson, L., Segal, J., Segal, R. (2021, September). *Emotional Eating – Help.* Retrieved December 2, 2021, from
https://www.helpguide.org/articles/diets/emotionaleating.htm#:~:text=Emotional%20eating%20is%20using%20food%20to%20make%20yourself,remain%2C%20but%20you%20also%20feel%20guilty%20for%20overeating.uide.org

Stanborough, R., (2021, January). *15 Non-Scale Victories to Celebrate for Weight Loss.* Retrieved July 25, 2023, from https://www.healthline.com/health/non-scale-victories#non-scale-victories-to-celebrate

Symptoms of PTSD in Adults (Plus Treatment Options). Betterhelp.com. Retrieved June 16, 2023, from https://www.betterhelp.com/advice/ptsd/22-symptoms-of-ptsd-in-adults/

Tanya Basu, *Why More Girls—and Women—Than Ever Are Now Being Diagnosed with ADHD*, New York, January 20, 2016. Retrieved April 10, 2017, from http://nymag.com/scienceofus/2016/01/why-more-girls-are-being-diagnosed-with-adhd.html.

The mental health struggles of weight loss surgery. Psychologytoday.com. Retrieved July 18, 2023, from https://www.psychologytoday.com/us/blog/the-truth-about-exercise-addiction/201611/the-mental-health-struggles-weight-loss-surgery

Top 10 Gastric Sleeve Regrets from ACTUAL Patients. Mexicobariatriccenter.com. Retrieved July 26, 2023, from https://mexicobariatriccenter.com/top-10-gastric-sleeve-regrets-from-actual-patients/

Trigger. GoodTherapy.org. Retrieved December 2, 2021, from https://www.goodtherapy.org/blog/psychpedia/trigger

What is gratitude? Verywellmind.com. Retrieved June 7, 2023, from

https://www.verywellmind.com/what-is-gratitude-5206817

What is trauma? Psychcentral.com. Retrieved July 13, 2023, from

https://psychcentral.com/health/what-is-trauma#definition

Why are vitamins important after bariatric surgery. Mayoclinic.org. Retrieved May 24, 2023, from

https://connect.mayoclinic.org/blog/weight-management-1/newsfeed- post/expert-answer-why-are-vitamins-important-after-bariatric-surgery/

www.ingramcontent.com/pod-product-compliance
Lightning Source LLC
Chambersburg PA
CBHW060822170526
45158CB00001B/53